"The day I read this book was the day I received my copy of the National Research Council's massive book *Diet and Chronic Disease* by a large group of the nation's leading authorities on nutrition and health. There are many similarities between what Dr. Davis recommends in ULTRAFIT and what the national authorities recommend."

—Norman Kaplan, M.D.,
from the Foreword

A unique new program of healthy weight loss and vibrant living, the Ultrafit program is a highly personalized plan that you can stick to for life. Now you can feel better than you ever thought possible. With Dr. Davis' revolutionary new approach, "ultrafitness" is finally within your reach!

JOE DAVIS, M.D., practices internal and preventive medicine in Texas. He graduated at the top of his class from the University of Texas Southwestern Medical School. He was also a teaching fellow at Harvard Medical and Massachusetts General Hospital. His hobby is competitive bodybuilding, for which he has won several championships. LUCILLE ENIX, an editorial consultant, has a B.S. in Foods and Nutrition and has completed a dietetic internship.

ULTRAFIT

How to Lose 5 Pounds in 7 Days Without Feeling Hungry

---

by Joe Davis, M.D., with Lucille Enix

With a Foreword by
Norman Kaplan, M.D.

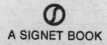

A SIGNET BOOK

SIGNET
Published by the Penguin Group
Penguin Books USA Inc., 375 Hudson Street,
New York, New York 10014, U.S.A.
Penguin Books Ltd, 27 Wrights Lane,
London W8 5TZ, England
Penguin Books Australia Ltd, Ringwood,
Victoria, Australia
Penguin Books Canada Ltd, 2801 John Street,
Markham, Ontario, Canada L3R 1B4
Penguin Books (N.Z.) Ltd, 182–190 Wairau Road,
Auckland 10, New Zealand

Penguin Books Ltd, Registered Offices:
Harmondsworth, Middlesex, England

Published by Signet, an imprint of New American Library, a division of
Penguin Books USA Inc. Previously published, under the title *The Ultrafit
Diet*, in an NAL Books edition.

First Signet Printing, February, 1991
10   9   8   7   6   5   4   3   2   1

 REGISTERED TRADEMARK—MARCA REGISTRADA

Printed in the United States of America

PUBLISHER'S NOTE
The ideas, procedures, and suggestions contained in this book are not
intended as a substitute for consulting with your physician. All matters
regarding your health require medical supervision.

*This book is dedicated to my patients,
without whose intimate sharing
of their lives none of this
would have been possible.*

ACKNOWLEDGMENTS

I wish to acknowledge the invaluable help of Diane Davis, who worked long and tirelessly in the preparation of the recipes and menus in the *Ultrafit* diet cookbook section of this book. My thanks go to Tom Davis and Bill Bosse, who gave me a gentle nudge and encouraged me to begin this book.

Contents

Contents for The Ultrafit Diet Cookbook (Chapter 8)

Foreword

The day I read this book was the same day I received my copy of the National Research Council's massive book *Diet and Chronic Disease* written by a large group of the nation's leading authorities on nutrition and health. As I subsequently read through that state-of-the-art analysis, the many similarities between what Dr. Davis recommends in *Ultrafit* and what the national authorities recommend in *Diet and Chronic Disease* became obvious.

A few examples will show the similarities:

♦ Cut down significantly on protein to no more than 6 ounces of meat a day

♦ Increase servings of fruits and complex carbohydrates

♦ Reduce markedly the intake of fat

♦ Increase servings of yogurt, cottage cheese, and other low-fat milk products

♦ Scrutinize food labels to know better what we are eating

The similarities go on and on. They demonstrate the first attractive feature of Dr. Davis's book: it rests on a sound base of nutritional and behavioral information. The second attractive feature is that it translates this sound advice into practical guides for all readers to follow.

I happen to be serving as vice-chairman of a committee of the National Research Council's Food and Nutrition Board that has been given the job of writing another book

showing the American public how to implement the basic
principles in *Diet and Chronic Disease*. I wish Dr. Davis
served on that committee. As I read *Ultrafit*, I marveled
at how much practical advice he provides to make it
possible for his readers to follow his program. He has
obviously learned what works and he describes these aids to
following the Ultrafit program in a remarkably straightfor-
ward and sensible way.

All in all, *Ultrafit* is an excellent book. Unlike many
diet and nutrition best-sellers, it is largely based on
sound scientific evidence. In a few areas, Dr. Davis goes a
bit beyond what is definitely proven, but I found nothing
that seemed potentially harmful in those few areas. Unlike
many diet books, it does not offend the intelligent reader by
offering impractical ways to reach impossible goals. Unlike
many diet books, *Ultrafit* will not frustrate the reader
by making absurd demands on either reason or practice. Dr. Davis knows who we are and how to motivate us
to follow a healthful life-style.

If you are concerned about your health—as all of us must
be—you will find a wealth of good advice and many aids to
help you follow that advice in this book. Better than
mother's chicken soup, *Ultrafit* can help us look and be
healthy.

—NORMAN KAPLAN, M.D.
Former vice-president
of the American Heart
Association

> The best men are molded out of faults and,
> for the most, are much the better
> for being a little bad.
> —VIRGINIA HADEN DAVIS

Introduction

Are you overweight? Do you feel tired when you get out of bed each morning? Do you take medications for chronic illness, such as high blood pressure, diabetes, heart disease, or arthritis? Are you unhappy with your sex life?

Do you feel tired before the day ends? Do you get frequent colds and the latest virus making the rounds? Do your emotions run from high to low without your knowing why?

If you have answered yes to two or more of these questions, then you and I have been down the same road. The first twenty-five years of my life I answered yes to most of these questions. The last fifteen years of my life, while studying and working as a physician, I learned that diet, exercise, and attitude could change my life as it changed my health. I found the Ultrafit State. I want to share that with you.

My discovery sounds simple, but it took a serious illness to make me realize my most valuable asset—my health. I want to tell you about that too.

I've always been an over-achiever. As a kid, though, I felt quite ordinary. My dad wanted me to play baseball, and I did, for him. After all, he had dreamed of becoming a major league baseball star. Perhaps he wanted his son to embrace the same dream. But my skinny body didn't allow me to achieve extraordinary feats. Never did I dream that I'd come to have a problem with my weight. My mom served me and my brother the usual meals all moms served their kids in our community: roast beef, chicken-fried steak, potatoes, gravy, cakes, pies, cookies. No matter what I ate, I never gained weight.

In college, I lived in the dorm and ate the food served there. I began to gain weight, but I felt pleased with my appearance because I began to look husky. In fact, I looked like a football player by the end of my freshman year. At the time, I thought of that extra flesh on my five-foot ten-inch frame as muscle. Now I recognize it as fat, and the beginning of my weight problem.

I always finished at the top of my class in college. I entered the University of Texas Southwestern Medical School at Dallas after three years of college, and without a college degree, because I ranked at the top among students. When I finished medical school, I graduated at the top of my class and received the most distinguished medical awards.

Then I entered my medical internship at one of the most prestigious hospital training programs in the United States—Massachusetts General Hospital in Boston. This became the most frustrating year in my life. Picture this. I had just spent seven years in school, making myself into my idea of the ideal doctor: technically and scientifically trained in one of this country's top medical schools. I planned to use these superior skills to serve and, yes, save mankind. Eight weeks into the reality of my internship, fear gripped my every action. What if a patient died on my watch? How could I make myself more alert and efficient when I only got to sleep a few hours every other night? Had I chosen the right profession? Did I want to minister to sick people all my life? To be responsible for their life and death? Every night I went home to my family, I drank myself into a stupor, trying to ease the pain of reality—the reality that I'd just spent a day trying to put patches on major illnesses. It seemed so senseless to try to put a Band-Aid over chronic illnesses that had developed over years.

As a physician, I had learned about illness. I had never learned about wellness. As the year progressed, I started to gain weight; my blood pressure rose; I felt tired when I got out of bed each day; I grew more and more depressed. I grabbed snatches of sleep and food when my work permitted. I did manage some exercise, usually at 4 A.M. in the living room while my wife and children slept. I ate and drank, like so many overweight people do, out of frustration, fear, loneliness. I began to lose touch with what makes us healthy. Finally, I got fat. At the end of my internship I weighed 220 pounds.

At this point, I questioned my choice of profession. I questioned my sanity. I questioned my ability to cope with my life.

Fortunately, an opportunity arose for me to work at the Heart and Lung Institute at Bethesda, Maryland, after I finished my internship. I saw it as a way out.

At that time, nine research units in the United States probed the problem of heart attacks. My work at the Institute embraced overseeing these projects. For the first time, I began to question why we, as a society, sank our resources into treating diseases that we could help to prevent. I began to feel hopeful that I could make my contribution by teaching people to take care of their *health*.

But, as usual, it took something more to get my attention. For all my over-achiever traits, I seem to be a slow learner. I contracted a severe case of influenza. Bam! It left me flat on my back for a week, and fatigued and coughing for several more. Performing physical tasks, easily accomplished before my infection, became a major effort and left me panting for breath at the end of simple things, such as walking to work.

The experience of the illness made me a more empathetic doctor to my patients, but it did more. I woke up!

I had been guilty of what the vast majority of us do. I had taken my health for granted. I had done just what all those very sick patients whom I had seen during my internship had done. They had made themselves vulnerable to chronic disease by ignoring their health until it was too late.

Suddenly I could see myself in them.

Because I had been studying disease, I thought disease represented a natural state in life. Disease is a reality of life. But health and vitality are the natural way of life. I realized that good health could be studied and understood just as disease could.

My true education had just began.

While at the Heart and Lung Institute, I became fascinated with nutritional biochemistry. This science concerns the interactions between what we eat and the many chemical reactions within the body. It was here I began to work on a dietary and exercise program that would produce super health.

Quite simply, I call this super health the Ultrafit State. The diet I created for all persons consists of a low-fat, low-protein, high-carbohydrate diet that I call the Ultrafit Diet.

At the same time, I became interested in bodybuilding as my hobby. I discovered that each of us needs an outlet to deal with the stresses of life. Bodybuilding gave me that, and provided the exercise necessary to maintain my health.

By the time I opened my private practice, I had learned that diet, exercise, and attitude had changed my life. I wanted to share what I had learned with my patients.

I saw patients with myriad medical problems. Once again, I came face to face on a daily basis with the hard reality that I treated patients with diseases that in large measure were preventable, if only the patients had eaten properly, exercised, and possessed a positive mental attitude.

As I tried to help others, I discovered a miracle. My own health improved! Helping others raised my own level of awareness, and I found myself moving toward what I now call the Ultrafit State. I had a constant supply of energy, I weighed in at my ideal weight—180 pounds, I enjoyed my family life each day, I felt good about my choice of profession and working with my patients every day. I no longer needed alcohol to ease the pain of living. Colds and viruses became a distant memory. And I began winning bodybuilding competitions. All these good things did not happen overnight. I evolved, just as you must evolve.

Throughout these experiences, I continued my medical training and research in health. I devised diet and exercise programs for myself, my patients, and my bodybuilding friends. During this work, I realized I had to find a way to help my patients from feeling hungry as I lowered the calories in their diets. I worked with a nutritionist/biochemist to develop protein and vitamin/mineral supplements to assist those with serious weight problems.

I am going to help you lose weight on less than 700 calories a day, without feeling hungry, while protecting your valuable muscle. The magic secret? Amino acids that control your appetite center while protecting your muscle tissue and helping you avoid the "yo-yo syndrome" of repeated weight loss and weight gain.

In addition to this Ultrafit Amino Acid Diet, I've devised another magic secret to weight control: the Pig-Out Meal.

This book represents the experiences of my patients and myself, working together to solve our problems and to sustain our attempts to reach the Ultrafit State, a reachable goal for each of you.

> Look to your health: and if you have it,
> praise God, and value it next to a good
> conscience; for health is the second blessing
> that we mortals are capable of;
> a blessing that money cannot buy.
> —IZAAK WALTON

CHAPTER ONE

The Ultrafit State

Congratulations! You have taken the first step toward your goal of reaching the Ultrafit State. What had seemed impossible will become a reality. On your journey you will become a more slender, vital, and energetic you.

The Myth of Variety

For most of this century, nutritionists, doctors, and teachers in the United States taught that everyone should eat a variety of foods each day: several servings of green leafy/red/yellow vegetables, three servings of animal protein, four servings of bread/cereal products, three/four glasses of milk.

How did the myth of variety get started? Until about 1930, medical research existed in a primitive state. Doctors had learned that lack of citrus fruit caused scurvy, that lack of vitamin D caused rickets. Beyond that, no one knew that much about the body's nutrient needs.

Doctors knew that if individuals didn't eat certain foods, disease resulted. In the 1930s, they learned that poor people who ate large quantities of single foods, simply because they had no money to buy other food, got diseases. The myth of variety began.

Doctors reasoned that if the lack of certain foods caused disease, then the safest diet should include a variety of foods. Who knew, the reasoning went, what other unknown nutrients foods might contain that the body needed?

In the 1970s, research available at the National Heart and Lung Institute revealed that if an individual consumed the variety of foods being recommended, that person ate too much fat, protein, and calories.

The result? People in the United States now face a different nutritional problem: premature death caused by heart disease and other chronic illnesses.

My work at the National Heart and Lung Institute taught me the fallacy in the variety of foods theory. If you eat the variety recommended for most of this century you will:

consume too much fat
consume too much protein
consume too many calories
consume too little fiber
make yourself vulnerable to premature death

The Ultrafit Diet cannot be described as a balanced diet, according to the variety of foods theory. I do not intend it to be balanced in that way. The Ultrafit Diet is balanced in regard to:

percentage of needed dietary fat
percentage of needed dietary protein
percentage of needed dietary carbohydrate
maximizing body muscle
maximizing metabolic rate

Let me repeat, the Ultrafit Diet consists of a low-fat, low-protein, high-carbohydrate diet.

The Right Ultrafit Plan for You

You will meet four people in this chapter. Each has her and his own story to tell. Each needed a different diet plan. You will see yourself in their stories, which will help you decide which Ultrafit Diet plan best fits you.

Three Diet Plans

There are three diet plans in this book. *The Ultrafit Amino Acid Diet* provides predigested amino acid tablets and vitamin/mineral supplements for people with serious weight problems who need help with hunger control. Don't let the word "predigested" scare you. Predigested simply means that the protein has been broken down to its most basic building blocks, those that your body itself breaks protein into after you eat it.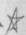

The Ultrafit Reducing Diet helps people lose weight more gradually. Just as does the Ultrafit Amino Acid Diet, the Ultrafit Reducing Diet protects your muscle and reduces the fat in your diet and on your body. This diet does not use amino acid tablets. It does require that you take vitamin/mineral supplements.

The Ultrafit Maintenance Diet helps people of normal weight who have health problems achieve that Ultrafit State. It protects your muscle as you reduce the fat in your diet and on your body. This diet includes a weekly "pig-out meal." The Ultrafit Diet Plans allow different people to eat the same foods, but at different calorie levels.

Edna and the Ultrafit Amino Acid Diet

Edna thought herself hopeless. She carried 265 pounds on a five-foot, four-inch frame. Edna had been sent to me by another physician as a last resort.

She had been on every diet ever invented. She suffered from diabetes, degenerative arthritis, and high blood pressure. She took four different medications for high blood pressure, one for diabetes, and two medications for the arthritis that racked her knees. She walked with a cane.

At age sixty-two, Edna finally got motivated. She knew a wheelchair or worse waited for her if she didn't change. Edna took the first critical step, just as you must. She committed herself to change.

In interviewing Edna, I learned from her experience on the numerous diets she had followed that she couldn't lose weight on 1000 calories a day. I recognized Edna as a slow metabolizer. I also recognized that her different diseases arose primarily from her excess weight.

If Edna could lose weight, her diseases would diminish. However, Edna had found that on a diet of 1000 calories or less she felt starved all the time and could not stay on the diet for more than two days at a time.

I put Edna on the 700-calorie Ultrafit Amino Acid Diet. I explained to her that the beautiful secret of the Ultrafit Amino Acid Diet lay in its suppression of her hunger. The amino acids, in tablet form, went directly into her bloodstream and tricked her brain into thinking she felt full. The amino acid tablets would help her maintain what muscle tissue she had and give her the needed energy to exercise, the other part of her Ultrafit program.

We had to design a special exercise program for her because of her physical limitations. Edna felt acute embarrassment about her appearance, so we had to tailor her exercise program to one she could perform in her home.

In ten weeks, Edna lost 48 pounds. Her body functions improved to the point that we discontinued her diabetes medication and all but one of her blood pressure medications. She feels better than she has in years.

Edna presents a special case in some ways because she suffers from several chronic diseases. She needs to work closely with a physician, as would any person with similar problems.

Louise and the Ultrafit Reducing Diet

I had been Louise's physician for nine years. She had always been faithful about coming in for her annual checkup. She enjoyed exercise and regularly walked or rode her bicycle so that she weighed, at age forty-eight, close to her ideal weight. Her clothes always fit her nicely.

Because of this I was quite surprised when she entered my office for her annual examination looking a little disheveled. She wore a loose-fitting tent dress, and the frown on her face in place of her usual smile told me something had gone awry in Louise's life.

She weighed 140 pounds, having gained 20 pounds since I had seen her the year before. Because of her small frame, five feet, four inches, she appeared to have gained more than she actually had.

During her examination, I found her body functions to be normal except for a borderline blood pressure elevation of 140/95, higher than it had been in the past. Her cholesterol had increased to 220, up from her usual 190. As I chatted with her during my examination, it became clear what had happened since I had seen her a year ago. Listen to what she said.

"Doctor Joe, this has been a rough year. My mother, to whom I've always been close, has been very ill this past year. She lives out of town and I've had to travel quite a lot to help my dad take care of her. I have really been stressed out.

"I found myself nibbling frequently, which is not my usual habit. I guess I got out of my routine. In addition, I ate out a lot. It was easier than trying to fix meals for Dad and me."

Looking back over her year, we realized it hadn't been huge amounts of extra food that had caused her problem. It was the day-to-day modest increase in fat in her diet that had caused her problem. The extra bag of potato chips here and there not only increased the fat in her diet but included extra salt. That had caused her blood pressure to rise. The evening handful of peanuts increased the same problem.

Instead of one glass of wine with dinner, Louise consumed two and three glasses. The extra wine seemed to ease the pain of living. The extra calories over the year had contributed to her weight problem in addition to aggravating her rise in blood pressure.

Louise did not have a history of weight problems and had not been on an actual reducing diet before. The 1000-calorie Ultrafit Reducing Diet fit Louise the best. This Ultrafit Diet, low in fat, and high in carbohydrates, would lower her blood pressure and cholesterol as well as her weight.

I gave Louise a copy of the same 1000-calorie Ultrafit Reducing Diet you will find in Chapter Six. I asked her to return for a checkup for her blood pressure, weight, and cholesterol every six weeks.

Three months later, Louise was back on the road to the Ultrafit State. Her blood pressure had returned to her usual 120/70, her cholesterol was now 180, and her weight had stabilized at a more ideal 120 pounds. Just as important as these numbers, Louise felt good about herself again. Her energy level had begun to rise and the characteristic smile had returned to her face.

Art and Charlie and the Ultrafit Maintenance Diet

Meet Art. As an accountant, Art sat behind a desk all day. He often worked fourteen to sixteen hours a day, propelled onward by his over-achiever complex. This left him almost no time for his family, friends, a healthy diet, or exercise.

Recently, I completed a physical examination of this forty-year-old man. At the conclusion of the exam, Art made this statement: "Doc, I don't know if you'll understand, but the other day, I suddenly became aware of a fact. For the last ten years of my life, it's not that I've been feeling bad, but I realize that I haven't been feeling good. Do you know what I mean?"

I answered Art: "I understand. Most people take their health for granted all their lives until something comes along that threatens their wellness. Or makes them aware of their lack of fitness to perform everyday tasks without pain or discomfort."

Art weighed 160 pounds, which was not too much for his five-foot, eleven-inch frame. His blood pressure read 120/70, which fell in the average range for a middle-aged man. His percent body fat ranged high at 20 percent. I showed him that I could easily pinch two inches of fat on each side of his waist. His cholesterol read 260 milligrams percent—high for Art's age. Art's other laboratory tests came within normal limits.

Art did not need to lose weight. He needed to lose fat. In reviewing his diet, I found Art needed to reduce the amount of protein he ate, particularly red meat.

Art needed to increase his intake of complex carbohydrates—whole wheat bread, potatoes, fruits, vegetables, cereal grains such as rice.

I gave him a copy of the Ultrafit Maintenance Diet (described fully in Chapter Seven). I showed him how to calculate the correct proportions of fat, protein, and carbohydrate his body needed. At the same time, I helped him understand that if he followed the Ultrafit Commandments of the Ultrafit Diets (page 107), he didn't need to worry about calculations.

No, Art did not need to count calories. He was fortunate. He needed to become aware that he could eliminate fat on his body by eliminating fat in his diet. The Ultrafit Maintenance Diet provides you with the principles for reducing the fat in your diet, increasing the complex carbohydrates, and rewarding yourself with the pig-out meal.

Art left my office with a prescription to increase his exercise as well until he could walk two miles in twenty-five minutes.

When I saw Art the next year for his annual physical, he had made considerable progress. He now worked a more reasonable nine-hour day; his blood pressure reading was

110/70—a better reading than before; his cholesterol had dropped a dramatic 70 points. We could find only one inch of body fat at his waist.

More important, Art felt good.

I used skin calipers to measure Art's percent body fat, but it can be determined by several other methods that I describe in Chapter Four. Once you know your percent body fat, you will learn if you share characteristics with Art, who carried his ideal weight but had too much body fat.

Everyone noticed Charlie's weight problem. I first met Charlie right after his twentieth birthday. He had just had his first attack of gout, a form of arthritis caused by high levels of uric acid in the blood. He had been taking medicine for high blood pressure, which interfered with his sex life, for two years.

Charlie worked as a carpenter when he wasn't ill with frequent colds and sinus infections. I knew his family history because his parents, my patients too, suffered from diabetes, high blood pressure, and heart disease. Charlie was setting himself up for an early death.

In the eight years I treated Charlie, I failed to persuade him to lose weight. He carried 270 pounds, much of it draped over his belt. His body fat measured an astounding 37 percent, and his cholesterol count was 320 milligrams, twice what it should have been.

One day Charlie's five-year-old daughter, the love of his life, asked, "Daddy, do you really want to look like a slob?"

That remark changed Charlie's life.

Suddenly he could now hear what I had been telling him for eight years. I put him on the Ultrafit Maintenance Diet that contains 2500 calories a day. For Charlie, this became a reducing diet. It seems impossible to most of us that anyone could lose weight on 2500 calories a day. That's the beauty of the Ultrafit Diet Plans. The Ultrafit Reducing and Maintenance Diets reduce the fat in your diet, use complex carbohydrate foods, and introduce an exercise program.

Within sixty days, Charlie had lost 42 pounds. His cholesterol plummeted to 190 milligrams.

Charlie's improvement sounds amazing. But it becomes a common experience when you follow the Ultrafit Reducing or Maintenance Diet plan.

Edna, Louise, Art, and Charlie represent the majority of my patients and, I believe, the total population. That's why I quickly sketched their lives for you. What they achieved, you can achieve.

In the following chapters, I will take you with me toward the Ultrafit State by describing the Ultrafit Diets. I will show you how they work, why they work, how you can learn to tailor an Ultrafit Diet to suit your special needs and life, and how you can devise your own exercise program no matter where you live or travel. I will provide you sample menus and food charts to help you get started.

If you commit yourself to becoming Ultrafit, I promise it will change your life. It changed mine. It changed Edna's. It changed Louise's. It changed Art's. It changed Charlie's. And it changed hundreds of others, including many of my patients'.

Attaining the Ultrafit State

You are starting a trip. Like any trip, you need to know where you are going before you start your journey. You need to know and understand the complete range of health states so that you can discover where your health falls. Only then can you start your own personal Ultrafit Diet program.

Step One: Know Your Body

Medical research conducted over many years with large population groups has shown that people who live healthy and long lives share known biological characteristics no matter where they live. While working at the Heart and Lung Institute, I studied these characteristics and came to think of them as important to the Ultrafit State.

Let's take a closer look at the physical and biological characteristics of someone in the Ultrafit State.

—You can walk two miles in less than twenty-four minutes, and still maintain a conversation at the end of your walk.

—You do not smoke. You limit your alcohol to no more than one and a half ounces of whiskey or six ounces of wine per day.

—You fall asleep readily at night. You get an average of seven to seven and a half hours each night.

—Your weight falls within 5 percent of your ideal body weight. I have listed these weights for you in Chapter Four.

—Your percent body fat falls in the right range. If you are a man, your percent body fat is 8 to 12 percent. If you are a woman, you have 15 to 18 percent body fat.

Step Two: Know Your Attitude

In my research, I learned that persons who share the Ultrafit State share certain mental attitudes. In the Ultrafit State, you should be able to answer yes to the following statements.

1. You are doing exactly what you want to do in life and feel generally happy.
2. You wake up each morning feeling great, not just good.
3. You take regular vacations.
4. You realize you are part of a large mutual support system and regularly offer your support to your family, friends, and colleagues.
5. You are committed to the basic value of life and see it as worth living.
6. You believe you have a mission in life, that your mis-

sion fits into a purpose that connects with the family of man in a larger universe.

7. You have a sense of humor. You can laugh at yourself when you find you take yourself too seriously.

Step Three: Know the Results

There are other ways you can know when you have reached the Ultrafit State.

First, you have taken charge of your health. You realize that, like illness, excellent health is a composite, made up of many different components. You recognize that you are responsible for those components.

Second, you have worked to make your immune system an ally. It is finely tuned, ready and able to battle infectious agents of all types, seeking out and destroying abnormal cells that could lead to such problems as allergies, arthritis, or even cancer. Colds become a distant memory. If you fall prey to one, it lasts only twenty-four hours instead of a week.

Third, you not only meet the average stresses of daily life head-on, you seek out challenges of your own. Even your vacations become physical challenges.

Finally, you have become an informed consumer. You carefully read the labels on all the food you eat and understand what those labels mean.

The Health Continuum

Your health can be looked upon as a continuum, or a road that goes from illness to Ultrafit. Now that you know where you are headed, let's examine some of the stages of this continuum more closely. How far along are you on the road to the Ultrafit State?

THE HEALTH CONTINUUM

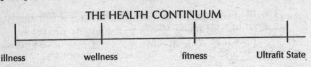

illness   wellness   fitness   Ultrafit State

Illness. Most people, including you, know that they lack health when they become ill. Illnesses that excess body fat can trigger range from the common cold to more serious problems such as a stroke or a malignancy.

Like Edna, people in this state become rather easy to motivate to change their health. They feel so uncomfortable they want to change. They listen! However, sometimes it takes a little reminding, depending on the degree of denial present.

Physicians like myself have spent the largest part of our time dealing with this illness phase of the continuum.

Fitness. Fitness implies wellness but includes more. Fitness means having the ability to withstand the normal or average stresses of daily living without symptoms.

If, for example, the elevator is out of order and you must climb the stairs, you are fit if you can climb the three flights without stopping to catch your breath and you don't feel your pulse pounding in your temples at the third floor.

If, for example, your son wants to play a game of catch with you, you don't need to cry for help to get out of bed the next morning should you say yes.

Or let's say your boss informs you that those construction reports are due in three days. If you are fit, not only will you be able to meet those demands, but you won't need to resort to several alcoholic drinks to help you relax in the evening after working on the project all day.

In the fitness stage of your health, you not only no longer take your health for granted, you actually take an interest in maintaining it. If, for example, your doctor tells you your cholesterol is high, you take the first steps toward eliminating some of those fried foods and dairy products you've been eating since childhood.

You exercise regularly, walking each evening with your

spouse, or by yourself. Interestingly, but not surprisingly, you have fewer and fewer lapses to the illness phase.

Colds may come, but they do not debilitate you as they once did.

Those tension headaches that once plagued you now grow more and more infrequent.

Most people who feel no pain or discomfort consider themselves well. I find these people particularly hard to motivate to change bad habits. Usually, you will not find symptoms in yourself from weight problems per se. But damage to vital organs may be taking place at such a slow rate that no obvious symptoms can be detected.

You may weigh 30 to 40 pounds above your ideal body weight. You may consider yourself "well." You don't hurt or feel uncomfortable. Like Art, you don't feel bad; neither do you feel good. Unfortunately, you have lots of company. Most Americans live in this phase of their health continuum.

Tragically, most Americans feel satisfied with this.

Because you've read this far, I know you don't feel that way.

Remember this. It's important to your health. Bad habits ultimately speed you backward toward illness.

Sadly, it often takes some time spent in the illness phase, as happened to Edna, to encourage people to act upon sound advice.

As I mentioned, it took a bout of influenza during my postgraduate work to awaken me to where I was on the health continuum. Until this episode, I, like the majority of Americans, had taken my health for granted. This marked the major turning point for me. I have since been on a journey toward the Ultrafit State, and I'm glad you have joined me.

Shortly, you will not only feel "well" most of the time, but you actually will begin to notice that you feel good. You will begin to discover that good health can be a powerful force, associated with positive feelings of well-being, rather than just an absence of feeling bad.

Finally, you will reach the Ultrafit State.

Your Ultrafit Body

—Your blood pressure is 100/70.
—Your resting pulse rate, taken early in the morning, ranges in the fifties.
—Your fasting blood sugar is 90 milligrams percent.
—Your cholesterol level reads less than 160 milligrams percent.
—Your triglycerides read less than 150 milligrams percent.
—Your uric acid is less than 5 milligrams percent.

You should know your percentages. If you do not, ask your physician. It takes only a small amount of blood to perform these tests. After you get your values, write them down.

Is Changing Your Diet Enough to Lose Weight?

True or false? People who have gained unwanted weight can lose it just by going on a diet.
False. No one can lose weight permanently without exercise and a positive attitude as well.

Nobody, my darling,
could call me
a fussy man—
BUT
I do like a little butter to my bread.
—ALAN MILNE
in *The King's Breakfast*

CHAPTER TWO

Fat: Your Enemy

It is my personal belief, as a physician of internal medicine, that dietary factors serve as the principal cause of our most common killers in the United States. The consequences of eating too much fat result in huge, staggering, burdensome problems. It costs society billions and billions of dollars each year to stem fat-related diseases.

Nationally, 32 million adult Americans, and a lot of kids, suffer in overweight bodies. Twelve million Americans are severely overweight. One third of all Americans go on some kind of diet at any point in time.

If you are overweight, you increase your risk for one of the following illnesses:

cancer of the colon
cancer of the breast
cancer of the uterus
cancer of the prostate gland
cancer of the lung
gouty arthritis
degenerative arthritis
heart attacks

high blood pressure
strokes
diabetes
suicide

I am not overdramatizing fat-related illnesses. Sure, other
factors figure into the equation that triggers any one of these
illnesses.

However, simply because you carry excess fat on your
body you increase your chances of developing one of these
illnesses in your lifetime. The longer you carry excess fat,
the greater your chances.

How Fat Increases Risks

The increased risk of cancer of the uterus or womb, cancer
of the ovary, and cancer of the breast in overweight women
relates to the higher estrogen hormone level seen in these
women. The female hormone, estrogen, stimulates cell division. The greater the rate of cell division, the greater the
risk that one or more of these cells will become uncontrolled
in its growth and result in cancer. Fat cells play an important
part in manufacturing estrogen. Fat encourages the production of estrogen: the more fat cells, the more estrogen.

The overproduction of estrogen hormone leads to excessive growth in the breast and womb tissue. Over a long period
of time, this can lead to cancer in these organs. If this sounds
grisly, it is. So is cancer.

This cancer is preventable. That's why I'm getting grisly
and technical with you. You must understand what excess
fat generates in your body.

Cancer of the colon relates directly to a high fat diet. The
higher the fat intake, the more likely you are to produce
toxic free radicals. Toxic free radicals exist everywhere, in
the air, earth, and our bodies. These free radicals (discussed
more fully in Chapter Twelve) damage the genetic code that

controls cell growth within the cells lining the colon. The uncontrolled growth of cells results in cancer.

High fat intake causes an increased secretion of bile acids. Your body produces bile acids to help you digest fats. Research studies show that bile acids produce tumors in the colon by increasing the rate of cell growth of cells lining the colon.

These statistics tell it all. Women and men suffer from colon cancer more than any other cancer.

Forty percent of all Americans will die of heart disease. Next to smoking, elevated cholesterol remains the leading risk factor for the development of heart disease. Excess fat in the diet serves as the leading cause of elevated cholesterol.

Why People Become Fat

In the past, everyone and everything seems to have received the blame for the high incidence of obesity in the United States. The real reason can be found if you look at the big picture; the time from the beginning of life on earth to the present. The answer lies in evolution.

The human animal has evolved genetic machinery for conserving and storing calories as fat during intermittent periods when food is lacking. Only since the twentieth century have we developed the technology for food production, storage, and distribution so that, for practical purposes, we no longer suffer from a lack of food—or at least not in affluent parts of the world.

Think about that. For millions of years, man constantly searched for food, suffered famines. Suddenly, in the last fifty years, the United States suffers from excess food production.

It takes work not to become fat in America!

Man evolved genetic machinery for conserving fat stores, the ultimate fate of all excess food, to protect him during periods of want. Our society now produces and preserves abundant food. The result? Too many fat folks with too many fat-related diseases.

Simply said, excess food has become a selective factor *against* those with the DNA makeup geared to conserving calories.

This leads to another point about evolution. Some individuals have been blessed with good genes that store fat efficiently, while others have not. Unfair? Sure, it sounds unfair. But if you lived in drought-stricken Ethiopia, you'd feel grateful for your genetic evolution that caused your body to stockpile and protect your body fat stores.

Women possess the most efficient fat-storing capabilities. Women carry a higher percentage of body fat than men. This extra fat serves two purposes, both related to reproduction of the species.

Remember, the more fat a woman carries, the more estrogen hormones she possesses. Up to a point, this increased amount of estrogen helps a woman. Regular menstrual cycles and the ability to make mature eggs in the ovary are dependent upon an adequate estrogen level.

Too much or too little estrogen interferes with egg production. You can read that another way. Too much or too little fat on the body interferes with egg production.

My physician friends and colleagues, dealing with infertility, find one of the most frequent reasons for a woman's failure to ovulate comes from too much fat on her body and the resultant high level of estrogen.

A woman produces an inactive form of estrogen in her adrenal gland and ovary. This inactive form of estrogen must be converted to an active form. This conversion takes place in the fatty tissues of the body. The more fat a woman carries on her body, the higher level of estrogen she contains.

Body fat serves a second purpose for a woman: body fat aids a woman in her evolutionary role in feeding the young. A woman needs the extra fat to provide her the ability to make milk during times of food scarcity. To produce milk, a woman must have some body fat.

Fat Requirements

How much fat do you need on your body? If you live in a northern climate, or near the North Pole and don't wear many clothes, you need a lot of fat. Maybe that's why Santa Claus looks the way he does.

Fat serves as insulation that prevents the loss of body heat. When you don't have much insulation you burn more calories to keep warm. You must burn more calories to keep your body temperature at 98.6, and that adds up to more food you get to eat.

For a man, 8 to 12 percent of his total body weight should be comprised of fatty tissue. This appears to be the most healthy. A woman needs 15 to 18 percent for her optimal bodily functions.

The average American male carries 25 percent of his body weight in fatty issue. The average American female carries 30 percent. The most grossly obese person can carry 60 to 70 percent of their body weight as fatty tissue.

If you eat a proper diet, your body makes the appropriate adjustments for your percent body fat.

Why People Stay Fat

"Doc, I swear to you, that I'm telling you the truth that I don't eat very much. When I go out to eat with my friends, they can't believe how little I eat. And just look at how fat I am."

I have to admit that the first fifty times I heard this, when I started my medical practice, I tended to agree with some of my former professors who had taught me that fat people have good mental erasers for what they eat.

However, ten years of medical practice have shown me, and fortunately medical science has now proven, that my patients were not liars. They did not eat as much as normal-weight individuals eat. They were not gluttons.

The facts: only twenty-five percent of women who are overweight exhibit gluttonous behavior. That is, they eat more than normal-weight individuals eat. Seventy-five percent of women who are overweight do not eat more than normal-weight individuals.

The majority of men who are overweight are gluttonous.

As already observed, evolution influences a woman to use efficiently the calories she takes in, and to conserve the fat on her body. Once a woman gains excess weight, evolution and her genetics can cause her to retain the excess weight even though she eats fewer calories than her body needs.

I'm not discussing this to discourage you, but to give you an idea of how you got fat in the first place and now have a problem losing that weight.

The truly gluttonous, content, overweight person I find as an exception, not the rule, in my practice. I've discovered that these kind of people usually operate as a team. Let me use an example of the husband and wife team.

Personally, I dread trying to treat a fat husband and wife team. Why? Let me tell you about Paul and his wife.

Paul recently approached me about a problem he had. "Doc," he said, "you've got to help me with my wife. She's fat and just doesn't seem to care. She seems perfectly happy.

"I tried to get her to diet, but I can't get her interested. Can you help me?"

This fascinated me. Paul's wife, as it turned out, weighed 200 pounds. Paul weighed 275 pounds.

Neither stood very tall. Both had high blood pressure. In reviewing their health habits, neither enjoyed exercise, and they got their greatest pleasure watching the Houston Astros on television while they sat in their easy chairs eating ice cream. I learned they encouraged each other to eat.

Neither felt threatened in their relationship. Paul later confided in me that he felt that no one else would want his wife. Interestingly, when I interviewed Paul's wife in private, she said the same thing about him.

I knew that if I could not help Paul to see his own problem with obesity, I could never expect his wife to lose weight. To date, I have failed to get either to lose more than 20 pounds.

They sabotage each other. For example, each time Paul loses at least 10 pounds, his wife bakes him a cake to celebrate some "special" occasion. Unfortunately, Paul or his wife will probably spend time in the illness phase of the health continuum before I can get them seriously interested in weight reduction, much less the Ultrafit State.

Negative Reinforcement

Paul and his wife serve as only one example of negative reinforcement. I see examples constantly in my medical practice.

I've seen cases where a husband or wife encouraged a spouse to become and stay obese for reasons as individual as the couple. Parents frequently select a child to become the fat member in the family. This happens particularly to the youngest child in the family.

Most of the time, I see negative reinforcement in the form of well-intentioned friends. Fat people like other fat people. When one goes on a diet, the fat friends make it difficult for the person trying to lose weight.

Negative reinforcement happens in subtle ways. A fat friend tells a dieting friend, "You don't look like you've lost any weight." Or, "How long did you say you had to starve yourself?" Or, "We love you for yourself, not for how you look." Or, "The more there is of you, the more there is to love."

Sometimes I must recommend to certain obese patients that they think seriously about developing entirely new friendships during their weight loss phase.

Are You Really Fat?

Why is it important to understand body-fat types? Here, I'm not talking about the classic body types: ectomorph, endomorph, mesomorph. I mean body-fat deposit sites.

You need to know your body-fat type because you may carry your ideal body-fat percentage, but not like the way you look in the mirror. Different people carry their fat deposits on different places on their body.

Evolution, combined with your genetic makeup, determines where you store fat on your body.

Particular storage sites vary from individual to individual, in large part due to the cellular dictator DNA.

Body-Fat Types

In my medical practice, I have observed that women in particular fall into three different body-fat types: localized obesity, central obesity, generalized obesity. Listen to the stories of these women, each with different body-fat types.

Diane: Localized Obesity

Diane, at age 42, first came to me concerned about wanting to lose weight. She stood five feet, six inches and weighed only 120 pounds. She kept running her hand over her hips, saying, "I can't get rid of these saddlebags."

I asked her to describe the women members in her family. I discovered that her mother and two sisters all had the same body configuration: large hips, large legs, small waists, small breasts, and thin arms.

We measured her percent body fat. She carried 9.1 percent body fat, a percentage that fell below her optimal level. Fortunately, she still had normal menstrual periods. This indicated that she had not yet fallen in the danger zone of too little body fat.

I explained to her that the fat on her legs did not affect her health. She had a cosmetic problem. At this point, I felt it unwise for her to lose more fat.

If she felt dissatisfied with the way she looked in the mirror, she needed to visit a plastic surgeon. Diane and I talked about her body-fat type and how her type could affect her health.

Her body-fat type, in its extreme, goes by the name of steatopygia in medical science. You may suffer from this yourself, or know someone who does. These people carry huge fat deposits in their lower body, but almost none in their upper body. The health consequences to them involve only degenerative arthritis of the knees.

In my medical practice, I find that women with this body-fat type suffer the most from body image. They don't feel good about the way they look.

Rose: Central Obesity

Rose had a much different problem and body-fat distribution. At 34 years of age, Rose stood five feet, four inches, and weighed 160 pounds.

Rose had central obesity: skinny legs, small hips, a large abdomen that measured thirty-three inches, which was four inches larger than her hips. Rose had large breasts and thin arms. She looked, in other words, like an egg walking on toothpicks.

We measured her percent body fat at 31 percent. Unlike Diane, Rose frequently skipped menstrual periods and had a problem conceiving a child. She suffered from diabetes and high blood pressure as well.

"Your body-fat type," I told Rose, "places you at high risk for endometrial cancer and heart disease, in addition to the illnesses you presently have." I ticked them off on my fingers. "You already have infertility, high blood cholesterol diabetes, and high blood pressure."

Rose's genetic makeup placed her at the greatest medical risk of all body-fat types. These people simply *cannot* afford to be overweight. Their excess fat compounds their genetic risk.

I explained to Rose that she could expect to be reasonably pleased with her appearance after she lost 35 pounds. Her menstrual periods would start regulating themselves and she stood a better chance of becoming pregnant because her estrogen level in her blood would fall.

Some women with this body-fat type, as they age, become stooped because the weight of their breasts pulls their shoulders forward and they generally suffer with the problem of stooped shoulders and back pain. Plastic surgery can help these women, by breast reduction.

Laura: Generalized Obesity

Laura, at 42, first came to me because she had pain in her knees. She stood five feet, five inches tall, and weighed 185 pounds. Fat covered her body like a blanket.

Laura had a fat face, fat neck, medium-size breasts, fat arms, fat abdomen, large hips which measured larger than her abdomen, and large legs. She told me how unhappy she felt about her life, her marriage, and her appearance.

After a physical, I found that she suffered from degenerative arthritis and high blood pressure. Her percent body fat measured 38 percent. In other words, she carried 70 pounds of extra fat on her body distributed in an even manner.

Laura had the most common body-fat distribution. Most men develop this kind of obesity. When these people achieve their ideal weight, they seem to enjoy their appearance more than the other two types, probably because the change is more symmetrical.

People with generalized obesity suffer from the same diseases as Rose, although they don't run the extremes in risk that Rose does.

Let me repeat. For optimal health, the Ultrafit State, I

recommend that men retain 8 to 12 percent body fat, and women keep 15 to 18 percent body fat. Genetics won't allow a man or woman with a big bottom to change that body shape. However, if that person carries the correct percentage of body fat, he or she will no longer place their health at risk.

Study your body-fat deposits. This should get you started analyzing your body-fat type.

Selective Fat Loss

Now look closer. Do you carry your fat saddles on your hips and upper thighs? Most people know their particular storage sites. I have, just as each of you, a "last fat stand" that depends on my genetics. I discovered this when I started bodybuilding. The last place I lose fat is the area under my arms at the side of my chest. I lose that last percentage of body fat for my bodybuilding competitions, but the loss does not enhance my health.

This leads me to a known fact in the Ultrafit State: *Not all weight gain is bad and not all weight loss is good.*

Let me use myself as an example. As a practicing physician of internal medicine, and as a competitive bodybuilder, I know that weight control, both weight gain and weight loss, plays an extremely important part in my life. Ironically, the focus on weight gaining, as a bodybuilder, led me to learn about the weight loss so important in the obese patient in my practice.

During the "off season" in bodybuilding, particularly in the early stages, a bodybuilder focuses on weight gain in order to increase the size of the muscles for the next year's contests. I gain weight by increasing my muscle mass while, at the same time, I retain my optimal percent body fat.

As I prepare for a bodybuilding contest, I strive to maximize my muscle mass and minimize my body fat. The reduction of body fat allows the muscles to "show through" the skin more readily. This process of losing weight, or "cutting up," taught me about safe weight loss. At this stage I can see my "last fat stand."

Notice that I only discovered my "last fat stand" *after* I reached my ideal body-fat percentage. Each time I lose the fat deposits under my arms before I enter a bodybuilding competition, I put my health in jeopardy because I carry less than my ideal body-fat percentage.

You cannot selectively lose body fat. I had to lose *all* my body fat before I could lose the deposits under my arms. I risked my health, too.

Look again. Do you have saddlebags? Do you carry love handles at your waist? Does your fatty site dimple—a condition known as cellulite?

Let's suppose you have love handles, and your fat dimples. At the same time, you weigh your ideal body weight and carry your ideal body-fat percentage. No matter how long you shake your body with a vibrator belt, no matter how often you cover yourself with body wraps, no matter how many "cellulite pills" you gulp, you will not get rid of your "last fat stand." Spot reduction does not work!

You can rid your body of its "last fat stand" only by putting your health at risk. If your "last fat stand" causes you to suffer severely from emotional stress, then perhaps you should visit a plastic surgeon to see if he can help you with the problem.

The Ultrafit Diets protect your muscle, reduce the fat in your diet and on your body, and provide abundant carbohydrate as the best source of fuel. Let me repeat: the Ultrafit Amino Acid Diet provides predigested amino acid tablets and vitamin supplements to help people with serious weight problems who need help with hunger control. The Ultrafit Reducing Diet assists people to lose weight more gradually. The Ultrafit Maintenance Diet helps people of normal weight, who have health problems, to achieve the Ultrafit State.

Now that you know the hazards of excess fat in your diet and on your body, I want to show you how you must use

your body and mind to lose that excess fat and reach the
Ultrafit State.

Myth: All calories are the same.
Fact: All calories are the same *in a test tube,* but not in
your body. Your body more easily *stores* calories contained in fat. Your body more easily *burns* calories contained in carbohydrates. That's why a high carbohydrate
diet is better for you.

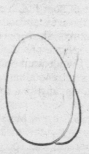

It is better to walk in the field for health
unbought than to sue the doctor
for a nauseous draught.
—BENJAMIN FRANKLIN

CHAPTER THREE

Using Your Body
and Mind
to Shed Weight

My patients give me all kinds of excuses why they cannot change their diet, exercise habits, and attitudes. They use their family demands, work demands, and, finally, their inherited genes.

When you decide to reach for the Ultrafit State, you must commit yourself to a life process. This means knowing your body and deciding to take charge of your life. You can use your body and mind to get rid of those excess pounds of fat.

Marsha serves as a perfect example. She brought her overweight daughter, Sandra, in to see me one day. She said to me in front of Sandra, "Doc, I don't want Sandra to be fat like me. Her grandmother was fat, and all my sisters are fat. It runs in the family. Can do you anything to help her, or is it just bad genes?"

"I can't give Sandra new parents," I told Marsha, "but I can help her to understand why her genes make her use calories more efficiently than other women. Too efficiently. She stores any excess calories as fat, rather than burning calories as a normal metabolizing woman."

In thirty minutes, I explained to Sandra how her DNA code dictated the way her body used calories, determined how fast she burned them, directed where she stored her excess fat, and how, knowing all these factors, we could help her lose that fat and keep it off.

Your DNA Dictator

For years, most physicians felt that overweight people had good mental erasers when they recalled what they had eaten. Many physicians still believe you become overweight only by eating more than normal-weight individuals. In other words, fat people eat in a gluttonous way.

Ten years of medical practice have taught me that the majority of women I take care of are not liars and really don't eat excessively. You'll be happy to know that "science," too, has proven that the majority of women are not liars about their food intake.

Instead, the answer (notice I did not say fault) lies in that mysterious but all-controlling cellular dictator, DNA.

DNA (deoxyribonucleic acid) is the chemical compound that our genes, or chromosomes, are made of. Biologically, DNA is the most important substance controlling all our body processes. Not only does it determine the color of our eyes and hair, it controls the production of every enzyme and cell in our body. DNA is located in the nucleus of all cells, and in our mitochondria, the energy-burning units in all cells.

It controls, in many instances, how fat we are or how fat we can become. It determines the rate at which we burn calories, and where we store those calories we don't burn. In other words, it determines where we store our excess fat.

Although DNA is the final regulator of all our body processes, it can be and is influenced by external factors. Exercise can and does signal the manufacture of more energy-burning units, the mitochondria.

DNA does this by sending out a messenger chemical called messenger RNA (ribonucleic acid). Messenger RNA causes proteins to be built inside the cell. Mitochondria are made from these proteins.

Although DNA may limit us in our goals, for the vast majority of us, our limits are usually taken from our environment.

Over a period of two years, Sandra came to understand the limits that nature placed in her body. But, using the same information that I will give you in this book, she is no longer fat like her mother and her aunts.

Sandra and I worked together to help her understand her friend, muscle, and her enemy, fat. Equipped with this knowledge, she calculated, just as you can, what worked best for her as she changed the negative image of herself with positive attitudes.

Your Best Friend: Muscle

In the war against our genetic fate, muscle acts as our ally. Fat, or adipose tissue, acts as our enemy.

Whether you want to lose 5 pounds or 50 pounds, want to become a bodybuilder like me or prepare your body for a beauty contest, muscle tissue and its content of mitochondria serve as your friend to help you reach your goal.

How many diets have you followed that focused on the loss of fat and paid little or no attention to the preservation of muscle? The Ultrafit Diet program, in any one of its three forms, is unique because it focuses on the preservation of muscle as the key to successful and permanent weight control.

One of the blocks Sandra had to overcome was her negative idea about building her muscle mass. She thought the diet and exercise program she selected would turn her fat to muscle and, although she would lose fat, she might appear more masculine.

Sandra's, or any woman's, hormones will not let that happen. The hormone called estrogen, made by the ovaries or taken in pill form, alters the way a woman responds to muscle building exercises.

Estrogen causes a thin layer of fat to be deposited underneath the skin, which smooths out any hard lines that might form, hard lines usually seen in a muscular male. If a woman drops the percentage body fat below the 15 to 18 percent recommended earlier, even she will begin to look hardened. Female bodybuilders that you might have seen on television or in the magazines have a percentage body fat of 4 to 5 percent, a level that I have already told you is not healthy.

Let me repeat: a woman always carries a layer of fat under the surface of her skin that softens the appearance of muscles. Men, because of their male hormone, testosterone, carry a thinner layer of fat just under the skin and thus appear more muscular.

Men and women need muscles. If you plan to gain permanent control over your fat stores, you must build adequate muscle tissue and its store of mitochondria.

Your Powerful Mitochondria

Have you ever wondered why your temperature stays around 98.6, even when you stand in cold air? You've got your mitochondria to thank for this. Mitochondria, the fuel-burning units, fill the muscular system, a beautiful organ, rich in blood supply. Mitochondria are your furnaces where you produce energy. Instead of using wood, coal, or oil as a source of fuel, you use glucose (sugar), fatty acids, and occasionally amino acids as fuel. Heat results from this energy production.

Mitochondria exist in all body cells. Trillions of them fill the body, and the muscles, our skeletal and heart muscles, contain the most. You cannot see these small egg-shaped structures with the naked eye or the usual light microscope. You must use an electron microscope to see them.

Because the Ultrafit Diets revolve around the production of mitochondria, it's important you learn about them.

Mitochondria serve several functions within the cell. Their most important role, the one that interests us here, is the processing of foodstuffs, particularly glucose and fat, to produce energy for our working bodies.

They contain numerous enzymes, or chemicals, that make the burning of fuel easier. The great thing is that their number is not fixed but can vary up and down. Mitochondria can and do increase in number, in response to increased demands placed upon them.

Eating more food does not increase their number, but regular exercise does. I am talking about simple exercise such as brisk walking—say, two miles in thirty minutes. Just a simple walk three or four times a week will accomplish this.

As the body needs more energy, your cellular dictator, DNA, directs the cellular manufacturing system to produce more mitochondria.

The more mitochondria you have, the more calories you get to eat, and the more fit you become.

On the Ultrafit Diets, the more mitochondria you have, the easier it becomes to lose weight, and the more energy you will produce. You need to do your best to keep these units working and perhaps add a few. This is why a diet without exercise won't work.

How to Protect Your Muscle While You Lose Fat

Nutritionists and scientists know that if you do not get a certain amount of protein and sugar (carbohydrates) in your diet, the mitochondria start using the muscle that they live in to stoke the fires, and destroy themselves. This will happen no matter how much fat you have on your body or take in with diet.

The Ultrafit Diets make sure this never happens by supplying enough protein, but not too much. Most people eat too much protein and fat in their diet. Providing your body with more protein than it needs does not build more mitochondria and it can cause real problems.

My experiences in bodybuilding led me to discover this fact. For years, physicians, coaches, and bodybuilding instructors taught that if you wanted to build muscles, you had to eat a lot of protein. I learned that this is not true. In fact, too much protein is bad for you.

The large amounts of protein that you take into your body contain large amounts of acids. When your body breaks down protein, sulfuric acid and phosphoric acid result. These strong acids leach calcium from the bones and cause them to weaken. You can develop a condition called osteoporosis, a disease much in the news these days.

I know because I developed osteoporosis from taking in too much protein for ten years after I took up bodybuilding as my hobby. When I broke several bones while training for a bodybuilding contest, I knew something had gone wrong. That got my attention! I began to experiment with myself and my protein intake.

I discovered that as I decreased my protein intake, I increased my muscle size. Much to my wonder, I found I got to eat more calories. Best of all, I had more energy.

Principle One: Super Health Requires Less Protein

This discovery led me to the first principle of the Ultrafit Diets. Protein should not exceed 15 to 20 percent of any person's daily calories. Let me explain.

The average American consumes 3300 calories per day. Of those calories, 40 percent come from protein.

Here's what's wrong with too much protein:

Excess protein turns to fat.
Excess protein erodes bones.
Excess protein wrecks kidneys.

What it adds up to is that excess protein erodes your health. Now when I counsel patients I tell them, if you can do only one thing to increase your health, reduce the amount of protein you eat.

When you eat more protein than you need, your body finds ways of getting rid of it. Some gets used for energy, the rest turns to fat.

If you want to lose weight, you must realize that you need to eat only a small amount of protein to preserve your friend, your muscle.

How much protein do you need daily? An adult, a regular person, needs 40 grams of high-quality protein, or 60 grams of intermediate-quality protein. A 6-ounce can of water-packed tuna has 50 grams of protein. One half of a chicken breast has 25 to 30 grams of protein. You see, it does not take much food to meet your protein needs. But don't worry about these numbers now. The Ultrafit Diets provide the protein your body needs. You will find the grams translated into menus and foods in other chapters.

What is the best way to get protein without the unwanted fat? Amino acid tablets, which we shall discuss in the Amino Acid Diet in Chapter Five.

Principle Two: Super Health Requires More Carbohydrate

For the past five years, Sharon, a grocery store clerk at one of our local supermarkets, has appeared for her annual physical. When I first saw her, Sharon, at age 25, stood five feet, five inches, and weighed 125 pounds, her ideal weight. Each year she has gained a few more pounds. The last time she came in, Sharon turned her back to the scales, attempting to avoid the reality that she had gained thirty pounds over her ideal weight.

When I suggested that we needed to talk about her weight, she said, "I don't understand what's happening. I rarely eat bread, and *never* eat potatoes, but I keep gaining weight."

Sharon, like most people, didn't understand how the body metabolizes food. She thought carbohydrates were the enemy, instead of essential to good body function.

Here's why carbohydrate is so useful.

♦ Muscle requires fuel to generate energy.

♦ Carbohydrates represent the most efficient form of fuel.

♦ If you don't provide your body with carbohydrates, your body burns its mitochondria.

♦ If you lose mitochondria, you can't eat as much and stay fit.

When carbohydrates break down in the digestive tract, they produce glucose, the fuel the mitochondria need. Glucose suppresses your hunger center and turns on your satiety center in the brain, which tells you you've had enough to eat. Complex carbohydrates also provide fiber needed for proper bowel function.

Carbohydrates have gotten a bad rap in terms of weight loss programs. You need carbohydrates. Bread, potatoes, rice, pasta, beans, fruits, vegetables, and cereals all provide rich sources of carbohydrates. I've made them an integral part of the Ultrafit Diets. In fact, I recommend on the Ultrafit Maintenance Diet that you primarily eat carbohydrates, both the complex and simple. I've made it easy for you to discover your carbohydrate needs, and how to calculate your needs, in Chapter Four.

Bathroom Scales Don't Tell All

Until recently, most weight loss programs focused on the loss of pounds—as indicated by the bathroom scales. These programs gave little or no thought to the true nature of weight loss—whether the person lost fat or muscle.

The Ultrafit Diets focus on, first, the preservation of muscle mass; second, the loss of fat; and third, the loss of pounds as reflected on the bathroom scales.

The Ultrafit Diets strive to save your muscle by providing the necessary fuel in the form of carbohydrate.

The Ultrafit Diets strive to get rid of fat on your body and in your diet.

The Ultrafit Diets recognize that muscle weighs more than fat tissue.

The Ultrafit Diets allow loss in inches, while increasing muscle mass.

Sharon had put herself on diets. But each time she lost weight, she regained the weight. She thought if she ate a high-protein, low-carbohydrate diet, she could achieve permanent weight loss. That's where she failed.

As Sharon and I talked, she began to understand that her diet caused her body to burn her muscle for fuel. The less carbohydrate she ate, the more muscle mass she lost. Each time she went off her diet, she regained weight rapidly because she had lost her mitochondria, the calorie-burning centers of the body. Without her mitochondria to burn the food she ate, her body stored her food as fat.

The Yo-Yo Syndrome

Sharon suffered from the common yo-yo syndrome, frequently seen in people who diet often. I designed the Ultrafit Diet Plans to avoid the yo-yo syndrome and Sharon's dilemma. The Ultrafit Diets protect your muscle by providing your exact body needs for protein and carbohydrate.

Principle Three: Super Health Requires Exercise

Every person you have met in this book began an exercise program. Here's why.

♦ Exercise signals your mitochondria to start working.

♦ Exercise increases your metabolism, the rate at which your body burns calories.

♦ Exercise reduces cholesterol.

♦ Exercise improves your immune function, increasing your resistance to infectious agents and cancer cells.

♦ Exercise reduces blood pressure.

♦ Exercise reduces emotional stress by triggering the release of chemicals that act as natural tranquilizers.

When talking with Sharon, I learned that she didn't know the wonderful array of exercise programs available to her. She thought exercise meant running or lifting weights. It had never occurred to her that she could increase her metabolic rate and build mitochondria by walking briskly through the woods as the sun rises, climbing the stairs where she worked, swimming, riding a stationary bicycle while she watched the evening news, or walking rapidly while window shopping during her lunch break.

I pointed out to Sharon that she had no choice if she wanted to break her vicious cycle of weight loss and weight gain. She must exercise.

I asked Sharon to return in six months. When she walked into my office, I saw a completely different woman. She *looked* ten years younger. I asked what happened.

Sharon had discovered a secret. To achieve a goal, you sometimes must do something you don't enjoy doing initially. Sharon found that she likes to walk. Now, she looks forward to walking thirty minutes during lunchtime each day.

MUST EXERCISE TO DEFEAT FAT × YOYO SYNDROM

She loves window shopping, and now finds she saves money by walking rapidly past the window displays instead of browsing through the stores. She feels better, too.

If you make health a priority in your life, use your imagination about the forms of exercise available to you. If you have not incorporated exercise into your daily life, start now.

Principle Four: Super Health Requires Low Fat Intake

The last principle of the Ultrafit Diets may seem the most simple, but it becomes the most important. If you want to get rid of excess fat on your body, which leads to the Ultrafit State, you must get rid of the excess fat in your diet. Here's why.

- ♦ Excess fat causes cancer.
- ♦ Excess fat causes rapid weight gain.
- ♦ Excess fat causes heart disease.
- ♦ Excess fat causes strokes.
- ♦ Excess fat slows your metabolism.

Fat in the Diet

The amount of fat in your diet holds the key to reaching the Ultrafit State. You can achieve this state by following any one of the Ultrafit Diets. Here's how much fat you need, man or woman.

Ten percent or less of your total daily calorie intake should be fat.

This means that if you take in 1000 calories, no more than 100 of these calories should come from fat. Here, I want you to start thinking in terms of grams, though you can follow any Ultrafit Diet without tallying the grams of anything.

One hundred calories of fat equals 11.1 grams. I've listed the fat content in grams and calories in the Fat Awareness Table at the end of Chapter Seven to start you thinking about certain foods and the fat content in different-sized portions.

You keep your metabolism at its most efficient rate when you consume no more than 10 percent of your calories in the form of fat. When you increase fat beyond 10 percent, you slow your metabolic rate. You do not burn calories as efficiently. Here's why.

You've read this before, but it's worth repeating. Your mitochondria use carbohydrates, and the resulting glucose, preferentially, for energy. Fat must go through a far more complex metabolic reaction before it can be used by the mitochondria.

Your body prefers to store the fat you eat for future use during periods of starvation. Evolution and your DNA see to that.

Remember our friend Charlie? If you'll recall, Charlie's daughter motivated him to lose weight when she asked him if he always wanted to look like a slob.

After Charlie got serious about his weight, we talked about what he ate. Charlie actually ate three meals a day that contained normal-sized servings. But look at what he ate.

For breakfast, Charlie ate two fried eggs, two slices of bacon, and buttered toast. At lunch, because he had to eat rapidly to get back to his carpentry, he ate at his favorite hamburger joint where he consumed two fried hamburgers, french fries, and a milk shake. Sometimes he ate two brownies. For dinner, his wife tried to please Charlie by preparing his favorite foods: chicken-fried steak, gravy, fried potatoes, green beans flavored with bacon, rolls and butter. Charlie had a sweet tooth, so his wife usually served him a slice of pie or cake. Sometimes he ate peanuts while watching television or ate ice cream before going to bed.

Do you believe Charlie ate in an unusual way? Neither did he. What he and most people don't understand is that fat contains the most concentrated form of calories of all food. Ounce for ounce, fat contains twice the number of calories as protein or carbohydrate.

Once Charlie understood this, he began to eliminate the fat in his diet. He began to lose weight, too, by eating 2500 calories each day. He continued to eat bread, potatoes, vegetables, milk, and meat, but he no longer ate them fried and flavored with fat.

Charlie decided not to become another number in the statistics that reveal one of the great tragedies in American society: deaths and physical/emotional burdens that result as the consequence of eating too much fat.

Of equal importance, Charlie decided to take charge of his life, to become responsible for what he ate, his attitude, and his exercise program.

Taking Charge: It's Up to You

Mary, the mother of three and a devoted housewife, believed others controlled her life. This very bright woman, who taught science at a local high school, had come to me because the aching pain in her knee joints had become so great that she could no longer climb the stairs at school. The pain forced her to seriously consider quitting her job, a job she loved.

Mary weighed 201 pounds and stood five feet, six inches. The degenerative arthritis in her knees had already caused so much damage that the destructive disease could be seen on the X-rays we took in my office. Mary's excess weight had caused her degenerative arthritis.

I pointed out to Mary that unless she lost weight her degenerative joint disease would progress until she became bedridden or confined to a wheelchair. At that stage, surgically implanted metal joints offered the only hope for her to walk again.

Mary and I discussed the principles of metabolism and

percent body fat, and the correct diet components that I've already outlined in the previous pages. Mary grasped the concepts quickly. *But.*

"Doctor Joe," Mary said, "I know I've got to lose weight. I see what you're telling me is true. But my family literally screams every time I try to change the way I cook. My husband insists that he is a meat and potatoes man, heavy on the meat and light on the potatoes.

"He also insists that he can't live without his roasts, chicken-fried steaks and gravy and, yes, his desserts."

I had heard this same reply countless times before. I knew the words by heart. Does this story sound familiar to you?

Who has charge of Mary's diet and her joints? I don't. Mary doesn't. Her husband seems to be in charge.

Mary, obviously a bright woman, knew that I was telling her the truth. She knew the future of her health. Before she ever stood a chance of planning a weight reduction program for herself, she had to take charge of her life. She had to take charge of her health. She had to make changes in her life to accomplish this.

Before you become successful in your effort at weight reduction and achieving the Ultrafit State, you must realize who's in charge of your life. I know that seems obvious. However, the majority of us act as if someone else is boss.

I see this problem and its solution over and over.

Listen to Harold, who coughed in such racking spasms that he exhausted himself.

"Doc, I know I need to stop smoking but my boss at work is driving me nuts asking me to do more and more work in less and less time. The pressure at work makes me smoke."

Who's in charge?

Unfortunately, Harold's boss has assumed control of Harold's work and his health. Is this fair? Is this correct? Absolutely not. Harold must take control of his life and health.

Shirley, another of my patients, knew someone else had charge of her life—her children. Shirley needed to lose 25 pounds of fat. She and I had decided that the Ultrafit Reduction Diet best fit her needs.

We came to a stumbling block, however, when we tried to work out an exercise program for her. No matter which form of exercise I suggested to her, she always answered with the same reply.

Excuse "I don't have time. I have to get up at six to fix breakfast and lunch for my kids and get them off to school. My husband and I both work. We're saving my income to buy a larger, newer house. By the time I get home in the evening, and get my kids off to their various extra school functions, I'm exhausted and it's late, too dark to do anything outside. I don't have time."

I said, "Shirley, do you believe what I'm telling you is true? Do you understand what we've outlined?"

Relate She answered yes to each question. Then I asked, "Do you believe your health is more important than that new house?"

I had to convince Shirley that she had to put her health at the top of the list, in front of everything else. If Shirley's health continued to deteriorate, she would never enjoy her children or any material goods she and her husband might buy.

Not Mary, Harold, Shirley, or any one of us can afford to leave our well-being in the trust of others.

Practice Rational Selfishness

When I talk to my patients about rational selfishness, some misunderstand the concept of "looking out for number one." When misunderstood, rational selfishness can be misinterpreted to mean narcissism, a self-centered form of destructiveness.

What is healthy selfishness? Let me start by stating the extremes. A narcissistic person directs self-interest internally and focuses exclusively on that self. An altruistic person directs self-interest externally and focuses exclusively on others. Rational selfishness strikes a healthy balance.

Here, I'm talking about healthy priority goal-setting. I find that I have the most trouble with this concept with women. Why?

Women possess, through genetics, the mothering instinct. Unfortunately, too many women carry this characteristic to a destructive level. They put every person's needs ahead of their own without regard to the consequences.

This may be the toughest obstacle to overcome in your effort to achieve the Ultrafit State.

Let me use Shirley as an example. Shirley has three children and a husband, all of whom she supports emotionally as well as providing for their physical comforts. Shirley has a full-time job that, with transportation time to and from work, consumes ten hours of her day.

She gets up at 6 A.M., gets her children off to school, and leaves for work at 7:30 A.M. She returns home at 6 P.M. and by the time she cooks dinner and gets her family settled, it's 8:00 or 8:30 P.M. Rightfully, Shirley collapses in a chair, too exhausted to exercise.

Shirley is right. She can't add hours to her day. Shirley can either eliminate some activity from her day or enlist help from members of her family. Either way, Shirley must make time for herself. This is rational selfishness. This is a healthy kind of selfishness.

Shirley had to realize, just as you must realize, that the people around you will benefit directly from this "selfishness."

Since Shirley had only 25 pounds to lose and had no life-threatening disease, I did not feel it necessary that she quit her job. However, there are people to whom I've made that recommendation.

Shirley had to ask herself which choice she wanted to make. She decided to take charge of her health. She chose to loosen her total control over every member of her family. That proved to be Shirley's hardest task, letting other people in her family assume control over their own destinies.

After a family conference, different members of the family accepted household chores. Shirley taught her children to make their lunches the night before. Because they arrived home before her, they started dinner preparation.

To Shirley's amazement, but not to mine, the children enjoyed cooking and the independence they gained. Shirley started taking them to the grocery store to shop. She instructed them about her diet and that she needed to restrict fat in her diet. Her children became the most avid label readers and knew more about food content than Shirley and her husband.

This entire process started with Shirley placing her own needs ahead of her children's apparent needs. She learned rational selfishness and, in the process, she actually benefitted the very people she thought, at first, she had neglected. Shirley gradually lost her 25 pounds, and she and her children began a different relationship that provided them with dimensions of living they had never experienced before.

Shirley learned to set priorities. You must learn, too.

Setting Priorities

What goes on a priority list?

Health, family, church, work, money, friends, travel, education, social position. How many people do you know who have made a priority list?

As a practicing physician, I have observed that people who make a list of priorities are the most emotionally healthy. Those who make health their number one priority are the most healthy, physically and emotionally. Ironically, people who make health their number one priority are those who have nearly lost their health.

If you have never made a priority list, perhaps I can help get you started.

Let me give you an example. I treat several ministers in my medical practice. One minister, who heads the largest congregation in a community, weighed so much he looked somewhat like a large penguin.

I asked him to give me his priorities. He said, "Ministering to my congregation, of course."

If he dropped dead of a heart attack within a week, had he reached his potential? Had he fulfilled his purpose in life? What had he achieved prior to his sudden death?

Developing a philosophy of life is a healthy thing to do. It is a positive step for your mental and physical health. It helps you organize your thoughts and realize you control your life. That is why you must decide on the priorities in your life.

Here are questions you need to ask yourself.

♦ What activity each day occupies most of my time?

♦ If I died tomorrow, what would I regret most not having done?

♦ What activity do I enjoy most?

♦ Have I tapped my potential?

♦ How much money must I have to provide food, shelter, the basic necessities of life?

♦ What activity on my list could I give up and not miss?

♦ Do I have talents? Does it matter?

♦ Who are the important people in my life?

♦ What do I do each day that has a positive effect on my health?

This list gets you started. Each of you will add questions as you create your own personal list.

I hope that health is first on your priority list. It should be.

Myth: Muscles turn to fat when you stop exercising.
Fact: Muscles do not turn to fat. If you eat the same number of calories, but stop exercising, the calories get deposited as fat on your body.

No one is destined to remain fat. You may have a slow metabolism, but you can speed it up with exercise and by eating the right kind of foods—ones that are low in fat and protein, and high in carbohydrate.

> Have you been able to think out and manage
> your own life? You have done
> the greatest task of all.
> —MICHEL MONTAIGNE

CHAPTER FOUR

How to Decide Which Diet Plan Best Suits You

Let me make a distinction among the three Ultrafit Diets so that you clearly understand which diet fits you. Certainly, each person who experiences excess weight gain has an individual problem. In the larger society, though, we know that men gain weight due generally to gluttonous eating. Women generally gain weight because they metabolize food at a slower rate.

I created the Ultrafit Amino Acid Diet for slow metabolizing women, and normal metabolizers who want a rapid weight loss of 20 to 30 pounds without sacrificing muscle tissue. The Ultrafit Reducing Diet meets the weight loss needs for normal metabolizing women and men. It accelerates your metabolism and protects your muscle tissue while you lose excess fat. I've designed the 2500-calorie Ultrafit Maintenance Diet to suit gluttonous men who want to lose weight. The 1500-calorie Maintenance Diet also suits the normal metabolizing woman who needs to lose 10 pounds or who is at her ideal weight but needs to lower her percent body fat.

Before I help you decide which Ultrafit Diet fits you, let me tell you an important fact about any Ultrafit Diet you choose.

Mineral Supplement Needed

You must take a daily mineral supplement when you follow the Ultrafit Diets.

The Ultrafit Diets are deficient in calcium and iron. Most physicians recommend that women take a daily calcium supplement, regardless of what the woman eats. To make it easy for you to find your needs, I've provided this information in Chapter Twelve.

Know Your Percent Body Fat

When you follow an Ultrafit Diet, you need not carry a calculator or a slide rule. You do need to know your particular body needs to decide which Ultrafit Diet best fits you.

Although I say that you don't need to carry a calculator, I'm going to teach you how to calculate your percent body fat, how to determine your metabolism rate, and how to use a math formula to arrive at the number of calories of fat, protein, and carbohydrate your particular body needs.

Why?

You need to familiarize yourself with certain foods and their content of fat, protein, and carbohydrate. Just as you learn any skill, you first learn the specifics and, as you become more sophisticated, you can then follow general guidelines.

After you determine each specific, according to your body, write it down in the space provided at the end of this chapter. You will translate this information into a diet for yourself.

What Is Your Metabolism?

Each of you probably knows where your metabolism falls in relationship to others around you. You cannot calculate your own metabolism; a specially equipped medical laboratory can. But that's not necessary.

When I say that someone has a fast metabolism or a slow metabolism, what do I mean? The metabolism of the body means, simply, all of the chemical reactions of the body added together. Your metabolism represents a measurement of these chemical reactions, and is measured in calories of heat liberated during the chemical reactions.

You eat food and that food gets digested. Your body absorbs the digested food into the bloodstream. From the bloodstream, the nutrients travel to the cells of the body where they are used in the various chemical reactions. Overall, this is an inefficient system. Only approximately 50 percent of the food you eat is actually made into a chemical called ATP (adenosine triphosphate) that your body can use. The other 50 percent is released as heat.

Science has assigned the word "calorie" to measure this heat. When I refer to various foods as having so many calories, I am referring to their ability to give off heat.

When I say you have a fast metabolism, I am saying, in effect, that you burn up a lot of food for your size and, as a result, give off a lot of heat.

A person with a fast metabolism actually uses food inefficiently and wastes, in the form of heat, more of the calories than he or she takes in. The person with a slow metabolism is more efficient, and uses more of the food taken in for the chemical reactions of the body.

Unfortunately, one of those chemical reactions is the storage of fat. A person with a slow metabolic rate gets fat if given the same calories as a fast metabolizer.

Most women metabolize food slower than men.

Seventy-five percent of overweight women can depend on having the slowest metabolism of all persons.

Most men metabolize food at an average rate.

Fast metabolizers rarely become overweight. However, they too can suffer from overweight if they eat in a gluttonous way. They *can* become overfat without being overweight. Because fast metabolizers rarely become overweight, I have not included the caloric intake for fast metabolizers in the Ultrafit Height, Weight, and Calorie tables at the end of this chapter. I listed the caloric ranges for slow and average metabolizers because they make up the greatest number in our population and because overweight can be a problem for them.

The fast metabolizing man uses calories at the rate of 18 calories per pound of body weight per day.

The fast metabolizing woman uses calories at the rate of 15 calories per pound of body weight per day.

The average man metabolizes at the rate of 15 calories per pound of body weight per day.

The average woman metabolizes at the rate of 12 calories per pound of body weight per day.

The slow metabolizing man uses calories at the rate of 12 calories per pound of body weight per day.

The slow metabolizing woman uses calories at the rate of 9 calories per pound of body weight per day.

Look at the people around you. Look particularly for someone your own age and sex. Do you gain weight when you eat the same amount of food as they do, while they maintain their weight?

If you answer yes, and you're a woman, you should consider yourself a slow metabolizer.

If you answer yes, and you're a man, look again. Are you sure you ate the same amount of food? Ninety percent of overweight men have a normal metabolism. They just eat too much.

By now, you should be able to determine whether your metabolic rate is slow, normal, or fast. If you still feel unsure, talk with your physician about your metabolic rate.

No matter what your metabolic rate, you can carry too much body fat.

Calculating Your Percent Body Fat

Remember, you can find your percent body fat by using several different methods: underwater weighing, using skinfold calipers, or by using electrical impedance systems. A pinch test will not tell you your percent body fat. It can only give you a rough guide that you carry too much fat, something you probably know anyway.

You can learn your percent body fat at your local fitness center, the doctor's or nutritionist's office, or perhaps your local YMCA center. Or, at minimal expense, you can buy your own skinfold calipers. Skin calipers work by measuring the thickness of skin in various locations. By using a simple conversion table, you can relate your skin thickness to your percent body fat.

If you want to buy your own calipers, which I personally recommend, I included the address of one company for your convenience. The calipers come with body fat tables and illustrations that help you determine your percent body fat. Write to: Creative Health Products, 5148 Saddle Ridge Road, Plymouth, Michigan 48170.

To speed you on your way to selecting the right Ultrafit Diet for you, let me give a shortcut to determining your percent body fat. Look at the Ultrafit Height, Weight, and Calorie tables at the end of this chapter.

- ♦ If you weigh 50 pounds above your ideal body weight, then your present percent body fat is at least 45 percent.

- ♦ If you weigh 25 to 35 pounds above your ideal weight, then your present percent body fat is at least 35 percent.

- ♦ If you are a woman and weigh 10 pounds above your ideal weight, then your present percent body fat is at least 22 percent.

- ♦ If you are a man and weigh 10 pounds above your ideal weight, then your present percent body fat is at least 18 percent.

Remember our friend Art, the accountant, in Chapter One? He weighed 160 pounds, stood five feet, eleven inches tall, and carried his normal weight, according to our weight charts. Art did not feel well. I measured his percent body fat with skin calipers. He carried too much body fat, 20 percent.

What does that mean? It means that Art had 32 pounds of fatty tissue on his body. How did I arrive at that? The same way you can.

Here's the formula:

Total body weight × percent body fat = amount in pounds of fatty tissue.

Art weighed 160 × 20 percent (.20) body fat = 32 pounds.

How many of these 32 pounds of fat should Art keep?

The average man should carry 8 to 12 percent body fat.

In Art's case, we decided he should carry 10 percent body fat—10 percent of Art's 160 pounds equals 16 pounds of body fat—because he thought he could live with that. Did I recommend that he lose weight?

No! His weight was fine. But I did recommend that he lose body fat.

I suggested that he embark on an exercise program and follow the Ultrafit Maintenance Diet to increase his proportion of muscle tissue, while losing the body fat. Art did have a choice of losing the body fat without building his muscle mass. However, Art would have looked too thin, according to our society's cosmetic standards. Since the late 1800s, our society has encouraged men to show their manliness and wealth by developing muscular or portly bodies.

Here's another example. Dolores weighs 160 pounds and stands five feet, six inches tall. According to the weight chart at the end of this chapter, she should weigh 135 pounds, maximum. Does that mean she should lose 25 pounds? Not necessarily.

By using skin calipers, I determined Dolores carried 40

percent body fat. Let's follow our formula to determine how much weight Dolores should lose. Remember, not all weight loss is good, and not all weight gain is bad.

160 pounds × .40 = 64 pounds of body fat.

The average woman should carry 15 to 18 percent body fat.

Let's allow Dolores the full 18 percent body fat. To find it, take 135 (her ideal body weight) × .18 = 24 pounds body fat.

So she has 40 pounds of body fat to unload. Using these calculations, Dolores would weigh 120 pounds after she lost her extra 40 pounds of fat (160 − 40 = 120 pounds).

Dolores knew she would look too thin at 120 pounds. I told Dolores that, in that case, she needed to gain 15 pounds of muscle to reach 135 pounds. In summary, Dolores needed to lose 40 pounds of fat and gain 15 pounds of muscle to reach the Ultrafit State.

I realize that making these calculations can make you dizzy. Stay with me and you will gain a more solid understanding of the way your body works.

Write down your percent body fat in the space provided at the end of the chapter.

Calculating Your Total Calories

You need to know how many calories you will consume at your ideal weight. When you know this, you will know how many fewer calories you should eat if you need to lose body fat.

Look at the Ultrafit Height, Weight, and Calorie tables at the end of this chapter. Find your ideal weight and the range of calories you should consume, according to your metabolic rate.

In Dolores's case, she can consume 1400 to 1600 calories

when she reaches her ideal body weight and ideal body fat percentage.

This is important. Dolores kept a food diary and together we calculated that she consumed 1500 calories daily and she gained weight! What does that mean? It means she carried only 60 percent lean tissue, the tissue that burns her calories, whereas 82 percent of her body should have been lean tissue.

She needed more muscle mass to increase the mitochondria to allow her to burn more calories. *That's* why she must gain 15 pounds of muscle and lose 40 pounds of fat.

Dolores had a choice. She could follow the 1000-calorie Ultrafit Reducing Diet, or she could follow the 700-calorie Ultrafit Amino Acid Diet. Dolores chose the Ultrafit Amino Acid Diet (which is outlined in Chapter Five). Here's why.

Dolores could have lost weight following the 1000-calorie Ultrafit Diet, but she preferred to lose her weight more rapidly, yet safely. She planned to attend her high school reunion in four months, and she wanted to weigh what she had when she graduated. In either case, Dolores had to exercise to build her muscle mass and to increase her metabolism.

The mistake most people make is to look at those calorie charts and say, "I could lose weight by consuming that many calories." Not true. If a person carries excess weight, and a large portion of that weight is body fat, a lower calorie diet *alone* will not bring that person's weight down. Overweight people must build muscle while losing fat.

Write down your calorie needs in the space provided at the end of this section.

Calculating Your Protein Needs

Now that you know how many calories you need to take in to achieve your body weight and composition, I want to show you how you can determine how much protein you need.

Dolores lost her 25 pounds and improved her percent body fat to 20 percent in seven weeks on the Ultrafit Amino Acid Diet. I then placed her on the 1500-calorie Ultrafit Maintenance Diet. To help her understand her body's needs better, I showed her how to calculate her protein needs now that she weighed her ideal weight.

Let's follow Dolores as she calculated her protein needs, after she lost weight, to arrive at her 1500-calorie Ultrafit Maintenance Diet. Granted, she could have used the menus I prepared for this book (see Chapter Six), but she needed to gain some knowledge of her protein needs to enable her to create her own menus as a new way of eating. That's another reason you need to understand how I arrived at the protein percentages.

Women need 15 to 20 percent of their calories as protein.

Men need 10 to 15 percent of their calories as protein.

Dolores chose to follow the Ultrafit Amino Acid Diet because that diet contains 42 grams of the highest-quality protein known, and only 700 calories.

To arrive at the amount of protein Dolores can include in her 1500-calorie Ultrafit Maintenance calorie diet, here's the formula she used.

She multiplied 1500 calories × 15 percent (.15) = 225 calories of protein she should include in her diet daily.

Each gram of protein contains 4.5 calories.

To get the number of grams of protein she should eat daily, she divided 225 calories by 4.5 calories per gram = 50 grams of protein allowed on her diet.

$$\frac{225 \text{ calories}}{4.5 \text{ calories per gram of protein}} = 50 \text{ grams of protein}$$

Dolores and you can use the Calories/Protein/Fat/Carbohydrate/Content Table in the Appendix to translate grams of protein into foods you can include in your daily diet.

Calculating Your Carbohydrate Needs

To learn how to calculate your carbohydrate needs, let's continue following Dolores as she calculated her body needs.

Women need 70 to 75 percent of their calories as carbohydrate.

Men need 75 to 80 percent of their calories as carbohydrate.

To arrive at the amount of carbohydrate Dolores can include in her 1500-calorie Ultrafit Maintenance Diet, here's the formula she used.

She multiplied 1500 × 75 percent (.75) = 1125 calories of carbohydrate she should include in her diet.

Each gram of carbohydrate contains 4.5 calories.

She divided 1125 calories by 4.5 calories per gram = 250 grams of carbohydrate allowed on her diet.

$$\frac{1{,}125 \text{ calories}}{.4.5 \text{ calories per gram carbohydrate}} = 250 \text{ grams of carbohydrate}$$

Dolores and you can use the Fat/Protein/Carbohydrate Table in the Appendix to translate grams of carbohydrate into foods you can eat.

Calculating Your Fat Needs

To learn how to calculate your fat needs let's once again follow Dolores as she calculated her body needs.

Women and men need 10 percent of their calories as fat.

In the case of fat, you can drop your intake below 10 percent and remain healthy.

But, let's follow Dolores as she arrived at her fat intake needs in her 1500-calorie Ultrafit Maintenance Diet. Here's the formula she used.

She multiplied 1500 × 10 percent (.10) = 150 calories of fat she should include in her diet.

Each gram of fat contains 9.2 calories.

She divided 150 calories by 9.2 calories per gram = 17 grams of fat allowed in her diet.

$$\frac{150 \text{ calories}}{9.2 \text{ calories per gram fat}} = 17 \text{ grams of fat}$$

Refer to the Fat/Protein/Carbohydrate Table in the Appendix to translate grams of fat into food.

In all my years of medical practice, I have never seen a case of fat deficiency in the United States. In fact, two teaspoons of fat provide all the fat your body needs. Two teaspoons of fat contain 80 calories or, roughly, 9 grams of fat, or 5 percent fat in the diet. A diet containing less than 1 percent fat is simply not palatable to Western eaters. Eating less than 10 percent fat in your diet does not add to the health benefits. You reach a point of diminishing returns.

Ultrafit Assessment Record

Make your own personal record. This will help you decide which Ultrafit Diet suits you.

     205   Your Present Weight
     135   Your Ideal Weight
    Slow   Your Metabolism (Slow, Average, Fast)
?   50%   Your Present Percent Body Fat
     15%   Your Ideal Percent Body Fat
             (8 to 12 percent for men
             and 15 to 18 percent for women)
    1200   Your Ideal Caloric Intake,
             at Your Ideal Body Weight

Picking the Right Ultrafit Diet
for You

Next, I will help you determine which Ultrafit Diet best fits you. Use these simple guidelines.

Follow the Ultrafit Amino Acid Diet (Chapter Five):

—If you are a *woman* or *man* and your present weight exceeds your ideal weight by 50 pounds.

—If your present percent body fat exceeds 20 points above your ideal percent.

For at least twenty minutes every day, engage in some form of aerobic exercise (see Chapter Nine). Your body will adjust itself, building muscle tissue and losing the excess fat.

Follow the Ultrafit Amino Acid Diet (Chapter Five):

—If you are a *woman* and your present weight exceeds your ideal weight by 25 to 35 pounds.

—If your present percent body fat is 20 points above your ideal percent.

For at least twenty minutes every day, engage in some form of aerobic exercise (see Chapter Nine). Your body will adjust itself, building muscle tissue and losing the excess fat.

Follow the Ultrafit Maintenance Diet (Chapter Seven) that contains 2500 calories:

—If you are a *man* and your present weight exceeds your ideal weight by 50 pounds.

—If your present percent body fat is between 10 and 25 points above your ideal percent body fat.

For at least twenty minutes every day, engage in some form of aerobic exercise (see Chapter Nine). Your body will adjust itself, building muscle tissue and losing the excess fat.

Follow the Ultrafit Reducing Diet (Chapter Six) that contains 1000 calories:

—If you are a *woman* and your present weight exceeds your ideal weight by 20 pounds.

—If your present percent body fat is between 10 and 25 points above your ideal percent body fat.

For at least twenty minutes every day, engage in some form of aerobic exercise (see Chapter Nine). Your body will adjust itself, building muscle tissue and losing the excess fat.

Follow whichever 1000, 1500, or 2500 Ultrafit Diet is approximately 500 calories less than your Ideal Caloric Intake (see tables at the end of the chapter):

—If you are a *man* or *woman* and your present weight exceeds your ideal weight by 20 pounds.

—If your present percent body fat is between 10 and 20 points above your ideal percent body fat.

For at least twenty minutes every day, engage in some form of aerobic exercise (see Chapter Nine). Your body will adjust itself, building muscle tissue and losing the excess fat.

Follow the Ultrafit Maintenance Diet and consume your Ideal Caloric Intake:

—If you are a *man* or *woman* and your weight is up to 10 pounds above your ideal weight.

—If your present percent body fat is within 10 points of your ideal percent body fat.

For at least twenty minutes every day, engage in some form of aerobic exercise (see Chapter Nine). Your body will adjust itself, building muscle tissue and losing the excess fat.

Of course, different people have different sets of problems and become overweight for different reasons. It's my hope that one of the Ultrafit Diet plans fits you. I believe ninety percent of our population fits into one of the Ultrafit plans.

Each of you, eventually, will follow the Ultrafit Maintenance Diet. Begin to think of it as part of your life's plan.

ULTRAFIT HEIGHT, WEIGHT, AND CALORIE TABLES

Find your height on the chart. The first column to the right of your height tells you what your ideal weight should be. You've already determined whether you have a slow or average metabolism, so look to the right again under the column that gives your metabolism rate. That tells you how many calories each day you can eat to maintain your ideal weight.

ULTRAFIT

WOMEN

HEIGHT		IDEAL WEIGHT	SLOW METABOLISM	AVERAGE METABOLISM
Feet	Inches	Pounds	Calories	Calories
5	0	101–113	900–1000	1200–1350
5	1	104–116	900–1050	1250–1400
5	2	107–119	950–1050	1300–1400
5	3	110–122	1000–1100	1300–1450
5	4	113–126	1000–1150	1350–1500
5	5	116–130	1050–1150	1400–1550
5	6	120–135	1100–1200	1400–1600
5	7	124–139	1100–1250	1500–1650
5	8	128–143	1150–1300	1550–1700
5	9	132–147	1200–1300	1600–1750
5	10	136–151	1200–1300	1650–1800
5	11	140–155	1250–1400	1700–1850
6	0	144–159	1300–1450	1700–1900

MEN

HEIGHT		IDEAL WEIGHT	SLOW METABOLISM	AVERAGE METABOLISM
Feet	Inches	Pounds	Calories	Calories
5	4	124–136	1100–1300	1850–2050
5	5	127–139	1500–1650	1900–2100
5	6	130–143	1550–1700	1950–2150
5	7	134–147	1600–1750	2000–2200
5	8	138–152	1650–1800	2100–2300
5	9	142–156	1700–1850	2150–2350
5	10	146–160	1750–1900	2200–2400
5	11	150–165	1800–2000	2250–2500
6	0	154–170	1850–2050	2300–2550
6	1	158–175	1900–2100	2350–2600
6	2	162–180	1950–2150	2400–2700
6	3	167–185	2000–2200	2500–2750
6	4	172–190	2050–2300	2600–2850

It is believable because incredible.
—ROBERT BURTON
The Anatomy of Melancholy

CHAPTER FIVE

The Ultrafit Amino Acid Diet

700 Cal / With Predigested Protein
YOU WON'T FEEL HUNGRY

The Ultrafit Amino Acid Diet is a very low-calorie diet. I designed this diet primarily for people with slow metabolism who cannot lose weight on a 1000-calorie diet, for normal metabolizers who want a rapid weight loss of 20 to 30 pounds without sacrificing muscle tissue, or who want to lose 5 pounds in a week without getting hungry. It is safe. Even though you consume only 700 calories per day you won't feel hungry.

The secret to hunger control and to the effectiveness of the diet lies in the magic that amino acids work on your brain. To understand why this diet is so effective, let's look closer at amino acids.

All proteins—I mean all—consist of individual building blocks called amino acids. The term "amino acid" should not frighten you. In biochemistry we call them weak acids. They won't burn your skin or erode your bones and kidneys like sulfuric acid.

Amino acids make up all tissues in your body: your brain, heart, skeletal muscle, blood, and bone. Even the enzymes that help digest the food you eat are made of amino acids linked together in complicated fashions.

When you eat protein, your gastrointestinal system, even

the hydrochloric acid in your stomach, and the digestive enzymes just mentioned, break down the complex proteins you eat to individual amino acids.

In fact, the rate at which your body absorbs amino acids depends on how fast your body breaks food protein down in your stomach and intestines. It's important that your body have a constant supply of easily available amino acids. Here's why.

Amino acids control your appetite.

Amino acids build muscle.

Amino acids build mitochondria.

Amino acids stimulate your metabolic rate.

Once your body breaks down protein to amino acids and sends them into the bloodstream, the body sends some to suppress the appetite. The body takes other amino acids out of the blood and reassembles them into the huge number of proteins that compose your body.

Once your body has completed these tasks, it needs no more protein. Any excess protein is fated to cause bone erosion, kidney destruction, stored fat. This becomes your fate.

Kinds of Proteins

Your body requires twenty-two amino acids to carry on its dynamic growth and replacement. It can manufacture many of these. Yet it cannot make them all.

The ten amino acids the body cannot make, and must get through the food we eat, biochemists call essential amino acids.

It so happens that animal tissues and products like milk contain all ten essential amino acids. We consider them high-quality protein.

An egg white provides the highest-quality protein known to man because it contains the greatest concentration of the essential amino acids. Certain fish proteins fall close behind. Meat, milk, and cheese follow next.

Green vegetables, bread, corn, pasta, nuts, legumes like dried beans and peas, and potatoes have protein in them. We do not consider these high-quality because they lack one or more of the essential amino acids.

In simple terms, you must eat more low-quality protein to get the ten essential amino acids than if you eat animal protein. Exactly how much you must eat depends on your body size and individual needs. We don't know precisely how much. Nutrition is not that exact a science yet.

The Food and Nutrition Board of the National Academy of Sciences, the organization that dictates what and how much we should eat, doubles the average of protein turnover a day to arrive at a figure of 60 grams as the recommended daily intake of protein. Protein turnover means that protein which is broken down and lost from the body through the skin, gastrointestinal tract, and kidneys.

This 60 grams leaves you with a good margin of safety to deal with the varying quality of protein eaten. Remember, not all protein is the same. It takes more of a low-quality protein than a high-quality protein to replace the protein turnover just mentioned.

Predigested Amino Acids: The Protein of the Ultrafit Amino Acid Diet

One of the three Ultrafit Diet programs I call the Ultrafit Amino Acid Diet. The Ultrafit Amino Acid Diet uses a protein packaged in a different way: predigested amino acids.

These tablets have many uses.

- Bodybuilders use predigested amino acids to build muscle.

- Physicians use predigested amino acids to build muscle and tissue in burn patients.

- Physicians use predigested amino acids to preserve muscle in patients with kidney failure.

- Physicians use predigested amino acids to help heal patients after major surgery.

- You can use predigested amino acids to help you lose fat and preserve muscle and mitochondria.

I first became acquainted with predigested amino acids when I attended medical school. I first saw them used with Robert, a 26-year-old man who had Crohn's disease. His surgeon had to remove a large part of Robert's intestine because he had an obstruction. Without three fourths of his intestine to help break down protein to amino acids, Robert lost muscle tissue rapidly. We had to give Robert amino acids through his veins so that his body could repair itself.

Robert had to take predigested amino acids intravenously for the remainder of his life. At that time, it never occurred to me that I, too, would take predigested amino acids someday, or work with a biochemist to specially package them for bodybuilders and for my obese patients who needed help fast. They needed to control their hunger, and discover the magic secret of how that happens, which I will reveal in a few pages.

Again, I used my own body to test the use of predigested amino acids for bodybuilders. Here's what I did, and what I learned.

The Miraculous Results from Predigested Amino Acids

In medical school, I had learned that the growth hormone, located in the pituitary gland situated in the brain, stimulates muscle growth. I knew that vigorous physical exercise stimulates growth-hormone production. In theory, the more I exercised, the more growth hormone I produced, and that produced more muscle.

I knew, too, that amino acids provided the building blocks for muscle growth. Is it possible, I asked myself, to shorten the time to build muscle size by introducing predigested amino acids directly into my body immediately before I worked out?

I wanted to make my body more efficient, reduce my overall protein intake to the smallest amount possible, start the protein to working immediately, and reduce my calorie intake by eliminating the fat contained in food protein. The results pleased me enormously.

I increased my muscle size faster than ever before, and I reduced my body fat to the lowest in my life. When my bodybuilding colleagues witnessed my success, they asked me to help them. I began work with a biochemist to produce a predigested amino acid tablet that equaled the highest-quality protein available to man—egg white.

One day an overweight bodybuilder friend asked me to help him lose 25 pounds. I wrote out a diet for him that used all the principles I had learned about amino acids, body hormones, exercise, and hunger control.

In nineteen days he lost 25 pounds. He became so elated, he told all his friends, and then some. The next thing I knew, the local pharmacist started calling, trying to obtain quantities of the predigested amino acids for people who presented him the photocopied diet I'd written on a scrap of paper for my bodybuilding friend.

At the same time, I decided to place Marilyn, a 32-year-old mother of three, who weighed 224 pounds, on the diet I'd written for my bodybuilding friend. She had tried many diets before and now told me that she had decided to quit all diets. She'd decided her genetics predestined her size. She wanted to quit fighting.

I convinced her to try one more time. This time I'd help her control her appetite and calories with the tablets I'd tested on myself. I told her she would have to walk two miles each day, in addition to taking the predigested amino acids, and follow a rigid diet plan.

Two years later, Marilyn weighs 142 pounds. Not only that, she keeps her weight constant. If she gains 5 pounds, she returns to the diet that I have come to call the Ultrafit Amino Acid Diet.

Who Needs the Ultrafit Amino Acid Diet?

—Slow metabolizers who must eat fewer than 1000 calories per day in order to lose weight.

—People who cannot control their appetite and must lose weight.

—People who must lose so much weight that they need the encouragement of losing weight quickly.

—People who need to build muscle tissue while losing fat.

—People who want to lose weight quickly, while maintaining muscle tissue, to look good for an upcoming event, such as a wedding, graduation, anniversary, or reunion.

—People with adult-onset diabetes who don't need insulin but may be taking medication to control their blood sugar level.

—People who should follow a zero-fat diet, such as those with high blood cholesterol levels or high blood triglycerides, or with both.

A Unique Diet

What makes the Ultrafit Amino Acid Diet unique from any diet in the world?

This diet takes its protein from predigested protein that has been pressed into tablet form. Predigested protein goes directly into the bloodstream, bypassing the digestive process and becoming immediately available to the body.

When you consume less than 1000 calories a day, you place your health at risk unless you take three steps.

Step One: You must consume at least 40 grams of high-quality protein per day.

Step Two: You must consume at least 100 grams of carbohydrates per day.

Step Three: You must consume a complete multivitamin/multimineral supplement. How much? I've made this easy for you by creating a chart that shows how much of each vitamin and mineral your body needs. You will find this chart in Chapter Twelve.

The Ultrafit Amino Acid Diet takes each of these steps and safeguards your health while you lose body fat. No other diet can do this more safely.

A Thermogenic Diet

I call the Ultrafit Amino Acid Diet a thermogenic diet because it stimulates the mitochondria to burn more fuel. The fuel, in this case, is provided by your body's store of fat.

Scientists have long known that certain foods actually accelerate metabolism. Melons, berries, and protein make you burn calories at a faster rate. Predigested protein, in the form of amino acids, accelerates your metabolism without adding fat to your diet. If you get your protein in the animal forms, it has to come with fat, even chicken and fish.

Because predigested amino acids can go directly into the bloodstream, the protein starts working immediately to stimulate your metabolism.

Hunger Control

You cannot expect to control your weight throughout your life unless you understand what controls your hunger and your behavior toward hunger.

Your brain operates as a complex control center, divided into different areas that specialize, controlling your emotions, thoughts, and behavior. I'm interested in your eating behavior.

Just such a center controls your eating or, as medical researchers say when referring to the animal world, feeding. The body houses the center deep within the brain tissue in a gland called the hypothalamus. Control of hunger and feeding serves among the hypothalamus's most important jobs. All mammals have this center.

You can properly interpret the gland's importance by its location in the center of the brain, in a command control position. In this command center, researchers have found two subcenters. The satiety center finds its home in the inner part of the gland, while the hunger, or feeding center, finds its home in the outer part of the hypothalamus.

Scientists discovered that when they placed a tiny electrode in the satiety center and stimulated it electrically, the animal, if eating, stopped. As long as the electricity stimulated this center, the animal refused to eat and literally starved itself to death.

When scientists placed the tiny electrode in the hunger, or feeding center, and stimulated it electrically, the animal, if not eating at the time, started to eat. As long as the electricity stimulated the hunger center, the animal continued eating until it ate itself to death.

The opposite situation happens if you destroy or remove the hunger center; the animal refuses to eat and starves itself to death. Research has found that, by contrast, if you remove the satiety center, and leave the hunger center intact, the animal eats and eats and becomes progressively overweight.

What does this fascinating information have to do with the Ultrafit Amino Acid Diet?

You can control your satiety and hunger centers.

Controlling Your Brain

Your blood constantly bathes your brain, and the levels of sugar and amino acids in your bloodstream regulate these centers. When you elevate your blood sugar level and your amino acid level, you turn on your satiety center and turn off your hunger center.

I designed the Ultrafit Amino Acid Diet to maintain a constant level of amino acids and sugar to prevent you from suffering the usual hunger problems associated with a low-calorie diet.

Let me show you how control of your hunger is so important to your health.

Albert, age 70, had been my patient for three years. When his wife died of pancreatic cancer, Albert started gaining weight. His blood pressure started to rise, and his blood cholesterol rose to a dangerous level.

At one of his routine follow-up visits, I commented on his growing obesity, and his developing medical problems. He said, "Doc, I know I need to lose weight, but I seem to stay hungry all the time. Every time I get started on a diet, I do fine the first half of the day, but by evening I find myself alone and rattling around in that big house and I start to get hungry."

I suggested to Albert that many people with depression stop eating, but others go to the opposite extreme. I had to help Albert with his grief process over the death of his wife while at the same time helping him lose weight.

When he and I talked, I discovered Albert was a snack-aholic. He had to put something in his mouth all the time. The Ultrafit Amino Acid Diet was tailor-made for him. The exercise program we agreed he needed got him out of the house and walking fast early in the morning.

The Ultrafit Amino Acid Diet allowed him to put something in his mouth throughout the day, but he didn't have to cook special meals, something Albert didn't enjoy doing.

The amino acid and sugar level in his bloodstream kept him from feeling hungry.

When I saw Albert the next time, he wore a pair of suspenders to hold up his trousers. He proudly gripped the waistband and pulled out the slack and said, "Doc, my friends can't believe I've lost so much weight. I don't take the aminos all the time now. When I get hungry between meals, I just take about six of those tablets and eat a piece of fruit and I'm not hungry anymore."

Albert had lost 60 pounds in three months. His cholesterol level had returned to normal as had his blood pressure. More important, Albert began to make new friends and pick up his old friendships. He felt good again!

Eileen had a different problem. She had gotten so fat, and had been fat for so long, that her body contained almost no muscle tissue. Eileen carried 185 pounds on her five-foot, four-inch frame. Her percent body fat exceeded 48 percent. In fact, we could not measure her body fat with the skinfold calipers because they simply couldn't fit over the fat under her skin.

She told me she had followed every diet known to man and she could not lose weight, not only because no diet worked, but also because after two days she got so hungry she didn't care anymore how fat she got.

We talked about her specific needs, and I told her she first needed to gain muscle tissue before she could expect to lose weight. She actually yelled at me. "No way! No way!"

I had gotten her attention for the first time. We talked about the fact that she had almost no mitochondria, the calorie-burning units contained in muscle tissue. As long as she carried such a high percentage of body fat, she could expect to suffer hunger and continued weight gain even if she ate 1000 calories a day. I taught her the principle that fat people get fatter and skinny people get skinnier. The more fat you carry, the fewer mitochondria you carry to burn any excess calories. You will get fatter than a similar weight person with a lean body.

She promised she'd try the Ultrafit Amino Acid Diet for at least three months.

For the next three weeks from the time I saw her in my office, she called my receptionist each day, except on weekends, to announce, "Well, I haven't lost *one* pound!"

Then in the fourth week, she called and screamed into the telephone, *"I lost six pounds this week!"*

The next week Eileen lost seven pounds. The sixth week she lost seven more.

Eileen knew I had told her the truth. She had to first build up her muscle tissue, and thus her mitochondria, before she could lose weight, as measured on the scales. In the first three weeks, Eileen had actually lost inches, which puzzled her because the scales did not show any weight loss.

She had actually lost fat throughout the first three weeks while she built a store of muscle tissue rich in mitochondria. Her weight loss accelerated as she gained muscle tissue.

At no time, in the daily phone calls to complain about her lack of weight loss, did Eileen complain that she got hungry. Hunger, for Eileen, became something she could control with the amino acid tablets.

The See-Saw Problem

Over the years, the patients in my practice have taught me that when one of them followed a reducing diet, the person sometimes had more problems *after* the diet than before.

I call this the see-saw effect. Too frequently reducing diets do not provide the right combination of protein and carbohydrate to allow growth of muscle tissue rich in mitochondria. When the dieter returns to normal eating, he or she experiences weight gain. Why? No mitochondria stores.

Most people know this experience. This happens so frequently that the phrase, "I've gained and lost the same 100 pounds for years," has come into common usage. Once you understand how your body operates, you will know that when you lost the weight, you lost your muscle and what you then regained later was fat. That caused the see-saw effect.

Medical Cautions

The amino acid tablets used in the Ultrafit Diet program do not cause problems in themselves. However, any individual who reduces caloric intake to less than 1000 calories per day must take certain precautions.

If you have any medical problem that involves taking diuretics that deplete your body of potassium, you will need to have your blood potassium level checked at least once every two weeks while you're on the diet.

If you have diabetes and are currently taking medication for that disease, either in the form of pills or insulin, it is imperative that your doctor follow your blood sugar level. I have found that my diabetic patients who follow this diet have a marked decrease in their needs for medication.

In the case of a diabetic taking oral medicines, I usually see the patient's body change to the point that I eliminate the oral medications. In the case of a diabetic taking insulin, I usually see the patient's body change to the point that I decrease the dose of insulin needed. A diabetic must be followed closely. I ask them to come in about once a week while on the diet.

If you have a medical disorder of the esophagus, such as food sticking in your esophagus, that interferes with your swallowing, then this diet isn't for you.

Ultrafit Amino Acid Diet Principles

1. You must eat six meals each day.
2. You must drink six 8-ounce glasses of water each day.
3. You must take a carbohydrate food with each meal.
4. You must take approximately 7 grams of predigested amino acid tablets with each meal. Amino acid tablets come in different sizes. For example, if each tablet contains 1200 milligrams of protein, take six tablets six times each day. If you take amino acid tablets that contain 1000 milligrams of protein in each tablet, you take seven tablets with each meal. It takes 1000 milligrams to make 1 gram ($6 \times 1200 = 7200$ milligrams, or 7.2 grams).
5. Eat only the foods listed on pages 80–81.
6. Do not substitute any foods other than those allowed.
7. You must take a multivitamin/multimineral supplement each day. The chart in Chapter Twelve gives the correct amounts.
8. Do not skip any one of the feedings.
9. Every fourth week, rotate off the diet, using the Commandments of the Ultrafit Maintenance Diet, described in Chapter Seven.
10. You must exercise. At least four days each week you must engage in some form of aerobic exercise, such as rapid walking, for at least 30 minutes.

The Ultrafit Amino Acid Diet

Note: The following menus use amino acid tablets that contain 1200 milligrams of protein per tablet (a total of 36 daily). If you take the amino acid tablets that contain 1000 milligrams of protein per tablet, take seven tablets with each meal (a total of 42 daily).

Breakfast—Two slices of whole wheat toast, plus six predigested amino acid tablets.

Mid-Morning—Small apple, plus six predigested amino acid tablets.

Lunch—Small baked potato, plus six predigested amino acid tablets.

Mid-Afternoon—One orange, plus six predigested amino acid tablets.

Dinner—One ounce of high-fiber cereal with four ounces of skim milk, plus six predigested amino acid tablets.

Bedtime—One banana, plus six predigested amino acid tablets.

Substitutes. Each time you take the predigested amino acid tablets, you can choose from a limited number of foods. These include one of the following: apple, banana, peach, pear, orange, ½ grapefruit, 10 cherries, 10 grapes, 10 strawberries, 2 slices whole wheat bread, small baked potato, or ½ cup rice.

Liquid Supplements. Supplement your water intake with diet drinks, black coffee, unsweetened tea, or herbal teas. Drink no sugar-containing drinks!

Fats and Seasonings. Do not use any butter, oil, or dressings on any food eaten. Limit your salt intake.

Frequently Asked Questions

I've used this diet with hundreds of patients. They have questions, lots of them, and they ask the following questions most frequently.

Is this diet safe?

Absolutely. If you follow the Ultrafit Amino Acid Diet as detailed for you, and if you take the precautions for medical problems I noted, then the diet is absolutely safe.

Do I have to eat all the meals and take all the tablets, whether the number adds up to 36 or 42, and the vitamins and minerals?

Absolutely. You must not skip any meals. I've already explained the necessity of why you must take a vitamin/mineral supplement when you fall below 1200 calories a day.

How can I expect to feel the first day?

During the first few days of following the Ultrafit Amino Acid Diet, you may notice a little more gas than usual. This comes as a result of the increased carbohydrate load presented to your colonic bacteria. These bacteria ferment some of the unabsorbed fiber and give off hydrogen, carbon dioxide, and methane in the process.

You may experience a headache the first two or three days on the diet. The headaches should not persist. The headaches arise due to your body adjusting to a new caloric intake.

Is this a good diet for hypoglycemia?

Absolutely. Because of the frequent feedings of carbohydrates and amino acids, your body can control your blood sugar level more evenly.

What happens if I have an elevated cholesterol?

The diet, virtually fat-free, has a marked lowering effect on the blood cholesterol and triglyceride levels. I use it frequently in my practice to get patients started on a lipid-lowering program.

Can I make substitutions?

In general, I do not favor them. You may use the substitutions listed on the Ultrafit Amino Acid Diet. Changes encourage people to stray away from the program. If you follow the program exactly, you can expect satisfactory results.

Why are there no vegetables?

A big bonus of this program comes with its simplicity. It requires no significant food preparation. That means, do not add any vegetables. I have found that if I allow my patients to change this diet, they soon begin adding butter to their vegetables just to add flavor. The vitamin and mineral supplements provide your body with all its needs, including trace minerals, nutrients normally found in vegetables. The roughage in the diet assists you in bowel regularity.

My experience has taught me that if a diet gets too complicated, patients become discouraged and sometimes confused.

Can I substitute golf or bowling for the aerobic exercise?

No. These do not have enough uninterrupted aerobic activity to benefit your muscular tissue and their mitochondria. However, the sports do represent healthy recreational activities. Read Chapter Nine for the list of aerobic exercises and the discussion on the differences between aerobic and anaerobic exercise.

If egg white provides the most complete source of essential amino acids, why can't I eat egg white instead of taking all those pills?

You could. You'd need to eat the egg white of two large eggs with each feeding. One caution. The egg white requires digestion. The digestive process delays the delivery of the amino acids into your bloodstream and thus to the satiety center in your hypothalamus. Too, the digestive process prevents the total absorption of the protein, which means you will lose some of the protein. Those people allergic to total protein cannot eat egg whites.

For anyone who follows a 700-calorie diet, hunger control becomes critical. If you must wait for your body to digest the protein taken from a food source, your hunger center will signal your brain that food is in short supply and thus make you feel hungry. The amino acid tablets go directly into the bloodstream without having to wait for your body to digest them. They signal your brain that food is not in short supply, and you feel satisfied.

I can't swallow pills without gagging. Can you help me?

I find that people who have problems swallowing tend to tilt their heads back. That's the wrong physiologic position for swallowing anything. Tilt your head forward. Place the pills in your mouth. Fill your mouth with water and swallow.

I find that most people who say they can't swallow pills actually talk themselves into believing that. They don't want to swallow the *idea* of taking pills.

Are all amino acid tablets the same?

No. The amino acid tablets should be derived from the

predigestion of a high-quality protein. Casein, one of the main proteins in milk, serves as a common base of most amino acid tablets. This is a satisfactory protein. Egg albumin and lactalbumin also provide excellent sources of amino acids.

Read Chapter Thirteen, "The Informed Buyer." In that chapter I list distributors of acceptable products and discuss how to read labels.

Do not use a capsule that contains only a single amino acid as a substitute for a product that provides the ten essential amino acids in one tablet. For example, single amino acids, such as lysine or tryptophane, can be purchased in capsule form. Physicians use these single amino acids to treat medical conditions. They do not provide the complete proteins that your body needs.

What happens if I skip one feeding?

You may get *very* hungry. Here's why. The Ultrafit Amino Acid Diet uses two safe and effective appetite suppressants. Amino acids and complex carbohydrates that your body converts to glucose (derived from fruits and grains) reassure the brain that food is not in short supply, and signal the body to keep the metabolic rate at a higher level, luring excess calories stored in your fat depots and accelerating your rate of weight loss.

Because your brain does not have to suffer through wide swings in blood sugar or blood amino acid levels, you do not experience the ups and downs and cravings so common with most diet programs.

Learn About Yourself

The Ultrafit Amino Acid Diet provides another benefit. It helps you control your eating behavior by giving you clues. Stress, social interrelationships, and habit all influence your behavior. The improved sense of well-being you experience while following the Ultrafit Amino Acid Diet can lead you to an increased awareness of why you feel good, why you feel bad, and what you can do to control your feelings.

When you stay with the six-feedings-per-day program, the concentration on your diet helps you eliminate the mindless nonhunger habit of snacking that leads to downfall when following other diet programs.

How to Diet and Feel Full

The Ultrafit Amino Acid Diet uses two safe and effective appetite suppressants: amino acid tablets and complex carbohydrates. These reassure your brain that food is not in short supply and signal the body to keep the metabolic rate at a higher level, luring excess calories stored in your fat depots and accelerating your rate of weight loss.

How to Diet and Feel Energetic

When you eat too much meat, the excess fat in the meat breaks down only partly into ketone bodies. This produces ketosis.

♦ Diets that create ketosis make you feel tired.

♦ Enough carbohydrates in a diet prevent ketosis.

♦ Diets that provide enough carbohydrates give you energy.

♦ The Ultrafit Amino Acid Diet provides you with the necessary carbohydrates.

Too Many Vitamins/Minerals Can Make You Sick

Make sure that the vitamin/mineral supplement that you take when you follow the Ultrafit Amino Acid Diet contains *no more* than 5000 units of vitamin A, 800 units of vitamin E, 800 units of vitamin D, or 18 mg of iron.

When you purchase amino acid supplements, you must read the label carefully to make sure that you receive the amount of amino acids per day contained in 40 to 45 grams of high-quality protein. If the label does not state the grams of protein per serving, you do not want the supplement. Acceptable predigested proteins are: casein, lactalbumin, egg albumin. You can find what the ideal amino acid tablet contains in Chapter Twelve.

Remember this—that very little is needed
to make a happy life.
—MARCUS AURELIUS

CHAPTER SIX

The Ultrafit Reducing Diet

In Chapter Five we discussed the Ultrafit Amino Acid Diet that applies to slow metabolizing women and normal metabolizers who want a rapid weight loss of 20 to 30 pounds without sacrificing muscle tissue.

The Ultrafit Reducing Diet meets the weight loss needs for normal metabolizing women and men. It accelerates your metabolism and protects your muscle tissue while you lose excess fat. You will lose weight gradually while educating yourself to a lifetime eating plan. When you have lost the weight you need to lose, you can move on to the Ultrafit Maintenance Plan described in Chapter Seven.

Principles of the Ultrafit Reducing Diet

—The Ultrafit Reducing Diet contains the optimal amounts of fat, protein, and carbohydrate to maximize your metabolic rate.

—The Ultrafit Reducing Diet contains 1000 calories. But you do not need to count calories. I've done that for you in the menus (on pages 92–104) that give you a start in meal planning.

—The Ultrafit Reducing Diet works best when you follow the diet three weeks on and one week off. During the week off, follow the Commandments of the Ultrafit Maintenance Diet (on page 107).

—The Ultrafit Reducing Diet (like the Ultrafit Amino Acid Diet) requires that you take a multivitamin/multimineral supplement. You will find the daily requirements charted in Chapter Twelve.

—The Ultrafit Reducing Diet requires that you exercise 30 minutes a day, four days a week. Select one form of exercise found in Chapter Nine.

How the Ultrafit Reducing Diet Works

What makes the Ultrafit Reducing Diet different from other reducing diets?

In my work at the hospital and in my practice early in my career, I became disenchanted with the reducing diets I found my overweight patients following. Yes, the diets reduced the number of calories a person took in. At the same time, I found my patients consuming the same foods that created the medical problems in the first place.

Willie, a 63-year-old-man, had heart disease, diabetes, and elevated blood pressure and blood cholesterol. I had sent him to a cardiologist and, after catheterization, the consulting physician found that the disease had progressed to the point that nothing could help Willie surgically with his angina.

The cardiologist turned Willie back to me and said, "Joe, he's in your hands." I'd already given Willie all the medicines I could think would help him with the symptoms. Willie still had chest pains when he did such simple things as walking to the bathroom.

By now Willie had become depressed over his condition.

He thought his life hopeless. I felt otherwise. Willie needed to lose fifteen pounds. I sent him to the dietitian at the hospital who put him on the standard reducing diet recommended by the medical establishment.

I took a look at Willie's diet. Yes, the diet contained 1000 calories. Equally, the diet represented a classic example of the myth of variety. The diet contained the standard variety of foods, reduced in quantity. It didn't protect Willie's muscle tissue. It didn't reduce his fat intake.

What did the diet contain that I found so objectionable? Wieners, graham crackers, peanut butter, margarine, and beef.

I knew if Willie followed this diet, he could expect his heart disease to progress, and his diabetes to continue to give him problems. Willie became my first patient to follow the Ultrafit Reducing Diet.

I've since used this diet with hundreds of patients.

After six weeks of following the Ultrafit Reducing Diet, Willie had lost 8 pounds. More important, Willie's chest pains had disappeared. His blood sugar level fell into such control that I discontinued his diabetes medicine. His cholesterol level dropped 25 points.

With the reduction of his chest pain, he and I decided to increase his exercise on the treadmill and stationary bicycle. That was seven years ago. Today, Willie looks the vigorous man he is. I believe the Ultrafit Reducing Diet saved Willie's life. It certainly saved his mental attitude and gave him hope.

Is the Ultrafit Reducing Diet different? You bet.

Willie, and people like him who have special problems, demand different diets, diets special to them.

Vitamin and Mineral Supplements

Early in my medical practice, I scoffed at vitamin and mineral supplements. I had been taught, just as other doctors, dietitians, and health teachers, that Americans produced the richest sewage in the world by consuming vitamin and mineral supplements.

The facts are, vitamin and mineral supplements have their place. When Willie's intake narrowed to 1000 calories daily, he could not meet his body's vitamin and mineral needs. Nor can you or anyone else who consumes 1200 calories or less a day.

I put Willie on vitamin and mineral supplements. You, too, must take vitamin and mineral supplements when you follow the Ultrafit Reducing Diet. In Chapter Thirteen, "The Informed Buyer," you will find guidelines on how to buy vitamin and mineral supplements.

Ultrafit Reducing Diet Problems

Let me be honest. You will find the Ultrafit Reducing Diet has a certain sameness. You will find that you will feel hungry more frequently. If you value your health, you must make sacrifices for limited periods of time to reduce the fat on your body.

Vigorous exercise, for as short a period of time as 15 minutes, can help you control your hunger. Vigorous exercise releases adrenaline, which has a suppressant effect on the hunger center in the brain.

Vegetables that contain minimal calories can help in this way, too. For that reason, I created a list of vegetables that you can eat in unlimited amounts during meals and between meals while on the Ultrafit Reducing Diet.

Remember to avoid fats and oils in food preparation. Use spices and herbs for seasoning. Study the herb chart in Chapter Eight that shows you how to mix and match herbs with foods.

Unlimited Vegetable List

artichokes
asparagus
bamboo shoots
bean sprouts
beet greens
beets
broccoli
Brussels sprouts
cabbage
cauliflower
celery
chard
chicory
Chinese cabbage
collard greens
cucumber
dandelion greens
eggplant
endive
escarole
fennel
green, yellow beans
kohlrabi

leeks
lettuce
mushrooms
okra
onions
peppers: green, yellow, red
    bell, chili or banana
pickles (dill, sour)
radishes
romaine
rutabagas
sauerkraut
scallions
spinach
summer squash: yellow,
    crookneck, pattypan, spa-
    ghetti, scalloped
tomato (limit 1 per day)
turnip
turnip greens
watercress
zucchini

The three weeks of menus on pages 92–104 help you get started planning your 1000-calorie-Ultrafit Diet.

I want you to study the menus I've written for your Ultrafit Reducing Diet. Don't look at them just to see what you can eat. Study them to learn what *kinds* of foods you must begin to eat for life; look at how the foods are seasoned and prepared; think about the *quantities* of each serving.

Now I want you to turn to the next chapter and look at the Ultrafit Maintenance Diet menus. Notice that I've used the same menus for the 1500- and 2500-calorie diets.

Here's why.

You must wrap your mind around foods low in fat, high in complex carbohydrates. You must begin to think about eating *small amounts* four to six times a day instead of gorging three times a day.

In planning these menus for you, I didn't try to get fancy or try to fool you into thinking I'm some kind of gourmet chef. I planned them to teach you a new way of eating to help you reach the Ultrafit State.

When you study the 1000-, 1500-, and 2500-calorie menus, notice the differences in quantities of food, particularly carbohydrate foods. Pay attention to that. The quantities of carbohydrates increase, but not protein.

I find that one of the big stumbling blocks for patients who must change their diets comes in preparing foods for their families while one member must diet. I'm telling you that you can prepare the same foods and only vary the quantities.

As you learn to plan your own menus and prepare your foods in the Ultrafit way, you can draw on your imagination to add interest and variety. I've listed several cookbooks in the next chapter that you may want to read.

One last word about your Ultrafit Reducing Diet menus: as I explained, when your caloric intake drops this low, you must make sure you consume adequate protein to prevent muscle loss, and you must consume adequate carbohydrate to provide your muscles with enough fuel so they won't use themselves for energy. These menus provide adequate amounts of protein and carbohydrate to protect your muscle.

The menus also provide an ample amount of fat for your body needs. Before you read the menus, think about this important fact. *The total fat intake in your diet is much more important in determining your blood cholesterol than the cholesterol content in your diet.* Remember that we talked about your blood cholesterol, and that you need a low blood cholesterol count for your best health. Notice that the 1000-calorie Ultrafit Reducing Diet includes three eggs a week, more eggs than are usually recommended. I deliberately included three eggs to call your attention to the fact that you can take in more cholesterol safely when the total fat content in your diet is low.

You should eat *one serving portion* of each recipe called for in the menus unless I tell you to add more or less.

Sample Menus

1000 Calories

FIRST WEEK DAY ONE

BREAKFAST	½ grapefruit *Hot Oatmeal, served with 1 teaspoon brown sugar beverage of your choice
LUNCH	½ cup low-fat cottage cheese, sprinkled with chopped chives and parsley *1 slice whole wheat toast 1 medium orange beverage of your choice
SNACK	1 medium banana
DINNER	*Coq au Vin, served with 1 carrot, ½ medium potato tossed salad, seasoned with *Vinaigrette Dressing beverage of your choice

* I've included recipes for many of the dishes listed in the menus. These recipes are starred and you'll find them in Chapter Eight, "The Ultrafit Diet Cookbook." (The special cookbook contents page at the front of the book will help you find the recipe you want.) I've also included directions for cooking vegetables and for preparing salads in Chapter Eight.

FIRST WEEK   DAY TWO

BREAKFAST   ½ cantaloupe
*Herb-Scrambled Egg
*1 Bran Muffin
beverage of your choice

LUNCH   *Vegetable Poached Chicken Breast, served
with *1 slice whole wheat bread
lettuce leaves and tomato slice, seasoned
with *Herb Dressing
beverage of your choice

SNACK   1 medium pear

DINNER   *Shrimp Creole, served with ½ cup steamed
white rice
tossed salad, seasoned with *Vinaigrette
Dressing
beverage of your choice

FIRST WEEK   DAY THREE

BREAKFAST   *Hot Oatmeal served with 1 teaspoon brown
sugar
½ cup skim millk
beverage of your choice

LUNCH   *1 toasted Bagel, served with 1 ounce slice
Monterey Jack cheese
lettuce leaves and sliced tomato, seasoned
with *Vinaigrette Dressing
1 medium banana
beverage of your choice

SNACK   1 medium apple

DINNER   *Chicken and Pasta
                tossed salad, seasoned with *Cilantro
                Dressing
                beverage of your choice

FIRST WEEK DAY FOUR

BREAKFAST   ¼ cantaloupe
                *Spring Omelet
                *1 Applesauce Muffin
                beverage of your choice

LUNCH   1 medium baked potato, stuffed with diced
                steamed broccoli, seasoned with chopped
                fresh basil
                1 medium banana
                beverage of your choice

SNACK   1 medium apple

DINNER   *Mexican Chicken, served with ½ cup
                steamed white rice
                tossed salad, seasoned with *Cilantro
                Dressing
                1 medium orange
                beverage of your choice

FIRST WEEK DAY FIVE

BREAKFAST   1 medium banana
                ⅓ cup (1 ounce) bran fiber cereal
                ½ cup skim milk
                beverage of your choice

LUNCH   *Tuna Salad, served as sandwich with
                *2 slices whole wheat toast

lettuce leaves   sliced tomato
1 medium apple
beverage of your choice

SNACK 1 medium orange

DINNER *Chicken-Mushroom Cutlet
½ cup steamed parsley potatoes
steamed green beans, seasoned with *Herb Dressing
sliced cucumbers on lettuce leaves
beverage of your choice

FIRST WEEK DAY SIX

BREAKFAST ½ grapefruit
*Parsley-Poached Egg
beverage of your choice

LUNCH 1 medium pear cut in half, served with ⅓ cup low-fat cottage cheese with chives
2 rice cakes
beverage of your choice

SNACK 1 medium banana

DINNER *2 Chicken Enchiladas
tossed salad, seasoned with *Cilantro Dressing
1 medium orange
beverage of your choice

FIRST WEEK DAY SEVEN

BREAKFAST 1 fresh peach
½ cup low-fat cottage cheese, seasoned with favorite herb, ½ diced fresh tomato

*1 slice whole wheat toast
beverage of your choice

LUNCH   *Herb-Poached Chicken Breast, served as
sandwich with *2 slices whole wheat toast
lettuce leaves   sliced tomato
beverage of your choice

SNACK   1 medium apple

DINNER   *¾ cup Seasoned Pinto Beans
*1 piece Corn Bread
steamed yellow squash, seasoned with fresh
*Salsa
1 medium tangerine
beverage of your choice

SECOND WEEK   DAY ONE

BREAKFAST   1 medium pear
*Hot Oatmeal, served with 1 teaspoon brown
sugar
beverage of your choice

LUNCH   *1 toasted Bagel, served as sandwich with 1
ounce Monterey Jack cheese
lettuce leaves   sliced tomato
1 medium apple
beverage of your choice

SNACK   2 rice cakes

DINNER   *Stir-Fried Chicken, served with ½ cup
steamed white rice
tossed salad, seasoned with *Herb Dressing
1 medium banana
beverage of your choice

SECOND WEEK DAY TWO

BREAKFAST   ¼ cup (1 ounce) GrapeNuts with ½ cup low-fat vanilla yogurt
beverage of your choice

LUNCH   *Tuna Salad in lettuce cup
*1 slice whole wheat toast
carrot sticks *Vinaigrette-seasoned cucumber wedges
1 medium orange
beverage of your choice

SNACK   1 medium banana

DINNER   *¾ cup Turkey-Vegetable Soup
*1 slice whole wheat toast
1 medium apple
beverage of your choice

SECOND WEEK DAY THREE

BREAKFAST   *Cream of Wheat, served with 1 teaspoon maple syrup
beverage of your choice

LUNCH   ½ cup low-fat cottage cheese, seasoned with chopped chives
1 medium sliced tomato   green bell pepper wedges
*1 toasted Bagel
1 medium apple

SNACK   1 medium banana

DINNER   *Linguine with Clam Sauce
                tossed salad, seasoned with *Cilantro
                Dressing
                1 medium tangerine
                beverage of your choice

SECOND WEEK DAY FOUR

BREAKFAST   ½ grapefruit
                *Herb-Scrambled Egg
                *1 slice whole wheat toast
                beverage of your choice

LUNCH   *Turkey Burger, served with *1 toasted
                Bagel
                lettuce leaves sliced tomato *Vinaigrette
                Dressing
                1 medium banana
                beverage of your choice

SNACK   1 medium pear

DINNER   *Pan-Broiled Fish Filet, garnished with
                lemon slice
                fresh steamed asparagus, seasoned with
                *Vinaigrette Dressing
                1 medium baked potato, seasoned with
                chopped parsley
                beverage of your choice

SECOND WEEK DAY FIVE

BREAKFAST   ½ cup low-fat cottage cheese, with a twist
                of freshly ground pepper
                *1 slice whole wheat toast
                beverage of your choice

SNACK   ¼ cantaloupe

LUNCH   *Vegetable-Poached Chicken Breast, served
                 as sandwich with
                 *2 slices of whole wheat bread
                 lettuce leaves and sliced tomato
                 celery and carrot sticks
                 1 medium apple

DINNER   *¾ cup Split Pea Soup
                 *2 hot Buttermilk Rolls
                 cucumber slices on lettuce, seasoned with
                 *Vinaigrette Dressing
                 1 medium banana
                 beverage of your choice

SECOND WEEK   DAY SIX

BREAKFAST   *Hot Oatmeal, served with 1 teaspoon brown
                 sugar
                 beverage of your choice

LUNCH   *Tuna Salad, served as sandwich with
                 *2 slices whole wheat bread
                 lettuce leaves and sliced tomato
                 1 medium apple
                 beverage of your choice

SNACK   1 medium pear

DINNER   *3 Soft Turkey Tacos
                 (fill tacos with chopped lettuce and ½ diced
                 tomato)
                 1 medium orange
                 beverage of your choice

SECOND WEEK   DAY SEVEN

BREAKFAST
1 medium banana
⅔ cup bran flakes cereal
½ cup skim milk
beverage of your choice

LUNCH
*¾ cup New England Seafood Chowder
*1 toasted Bagel
carrot sticks
beverage of your choice

SNACK
1 medium pear

DINNER
*Baked Chicken Breast with ½ cup *Corn
Bread Dressing
steamed fresh green beans, seasoned with
*Herb Dressing
tossed salad, seasoned with favorite herb
vinegar
*1 Cinnamon-Baked Apple
beverage of your choice

THIRD WEEK   DAY ONE

BREAKFAST
*Parsley-Poached Egg
*1 slice whole wheat toast
beverage of your choice

LUNCH
*Vegetable-Poached Chicken Breast, served
as sandwich with
*2 slices whole wheat bread
lettuce leaves and sliced tomato
1 medium banana
beverage of your choice

SNACK   ½ grapefruit

DINNER   *¾ cup Chicken Soup with Rice
                  *2 whole wheat Muffins
                  bell pepper wedges
                  1 medium tangerine
                  beverage of your choice

THIRD WEEK DAY TWO

BREAKFAST   *Cream of Wheat, served with 1 teaspoon
                  maple syrup
                  1 medium pear
                  beverage of your choice

LUNCH   *1 toasted Bagel, served as sandwich with 1
                  ounce slice Monterey Jack cheese
                  lettuce leaves   sliced tomato
                  1 medium orange
                  beverage of your choice

SNACK   1 medium pear

DINNER   *Turkey Spaghetti
                  tossed salad, seasoned with *Cilantro
                  Dressing
                  1 medium apple
                  beverage of your choice

THIRD WEEK DAY THREE

BREAKFAST   ½ cup low-fat vanilla yogurt
                  *1 Bran Muffin
                  beverage of your choice

LUNCH   *Herb-Poached Chicken Breast, served as
                  sandwich with

*2 slices whole wheat bread
lettuce leaves   sliced tomato
1 medium apple
beverage of your choice

SNACK   1 medium banana

DINNER   *Creoled Haddock
⅔ cup steamed brown rice
steamed zucchini, seasoned with *Vinaigrette Dressing
1 medium tangerine
beverage of your choice

THIRD WEEK   DAY FOUR

BREAKFAST   ½ cup skim milk
½ cup bran fiber cereal
beverage of your choice

LUNCH   1 medium steamed potato, seasoned with
scallions
steamed broccoli, seasoned with *Vinaigrette Dressing
1 medium banana
beverage of your choice

SNACK   1 medium tangerine

DINNER   *Turkey Burger, served with lettuce leaves,
tomato slice, dill pickle slice
*2 slices whole wheat bread
*Fruit Salad
beverage of your choice

THIRD WEEK DAY FIVE

BREAKFAST   *Spring Omelet
*1 toasted Bagel
beverage of your choice

LUNCH   *¾ cup Split Pea Soup
*1 toasted Applesauce Muffin
carrot sticks   cucumber wedges
1 medium orange
beverage of your choice

SNACK   1 medium pear

DINNER   *¾ cup New England Seafood Chowder
*1 piece Corn Bread
tossed salad, seasoned with *Herb Dressing
beverage of your choice

THIRD WEEK DAY SIX

BREAKFAST   ¼ cup (1 ounce) GrapeNuts
½ cup low-fat vanilla yogurt
beverage of your choice

LUNCH   ½ cup low-fat cottage cheese, seasoned with
chopped chives and green bell pepper
*1 toasted Bagel
1 medium tangerine
beverage of your choice

SNACK   1 medium banana

DINNER   *Oriental Shrimp, served with ⅔ cup
steamed white rice

tossed salad, seasoned with *Vinaigrette
Dressing
1 medium pear
beverage of your choice

THIRD WEEK   DAY SEVEN

BREAKFAST   *Parsley-Poached Egg
                 *1 Bran Muffin
                 beverage of your choice

LUNCH   *Vegetable-Poached Chicken Breast
                 *1 slice toasted Buttermilk Bran Bread
                 lettuce and tomato salad, seasoned with
                 *Vinaigrette Dressing
                 1 medium apple
                 beverage of your choice

SNACK   1 medium banana

DINNER   *Orange Roughy à l'Orange
                 ½ cup steamed parsley potatoes
                 fresh steamed broccoli, seasoned with
                 *Herb Dressing
                 carrot and celery sticks
                 1 medium pear
                 beverage of your choice

Does the Ultrafit Diet Give You a Free Lunch?

Yes. Vegetables high in water and fiber (see the list on
page 90) can be eaten throughout the day without making
you gain weight.

Too Many Vitamins/Minerals Can Make You Sick

Make sure that the vitamin/mineral supplement that you take when you follow the Ultrafit Reducing Diet contains *no more* than 5000 units of vitamin A, 800 units of vitamin E, 800 units of vitamin D, or 18 mg or iron.

> Common sense is not so common.
> —VOLTAIRE

CHAPTER SEVEN

The Ultrafit
Maintenance Diet

I've designed the 2500-calorie Ultrafit Maintenance Diet for gluttonous men who want to lose weight. The Ultrafit 1500-calorie Maintenance Diet suits the normal metabolizing woman who needs to lose less than 10 pounds or who is at her ideal weight but needs to lower her percent body fat.

The Ultrafit Maintenance Diet will serve you well for the rest of your life. If you began your diet by following the Ultrafit Amino Acid Diet or the Ultrafit Reducing Diet, you eventually will find your way here. The Ultrafit Maintenance Diet helps lead you to the Ultrafit State. It maximizes your muscle tissue and insures that you maintain your best metabolic rate.

- The Ultrafit Maintenance Diet does not require you to count calories.

- The Ultrafit Maintenance Diet provides the best way to lower elevated blood cholesterol.

- The Ultrafit Maintenance Diet provides the best way to lower elevated blood pressure.

- The Ultrafit Maintenance Diet provides the best way to control diabetes that can be regulated by diet.

All your life you must stay conscious of what you eat.

You will be healthier and happier when you follow the Ultrafit Commandments. Don't feel put off by what may sound like dictatorial rules. Common sense lies behind all of these Commandments. My patients love them because the Commandments help individuals review their self-control.

Ultrafit Commandments

1. Limit your fat to 10 percent of your total caloric intake. You will not become fat deficient.
2. Divide your total food intake into four to six small meals per day.
3. Bake, broil, boil, or microwave your foods. Do not fry foods or coat them with batter. If you stir-fry, use a nonstick cooking spray, or use no more than one teaspoon of fat. I used to eat so many fried foods that a neighbor once asked my wife how she planned to fry the turkey for Thanksgiving.
4. Eat red meat no more than once a week, and then only if you feel you must.
5. Try not to eat pork products. That means bacon, ham, and all kinds of sausage.
6. Use skim milk only. Use caution when buying buttermilk. Be sure to read the label. You can depend on wholesome low-fat products only after the butterfat has been removed from milk. The label should read ½ percent buttermilk. Don't accept anything higher.
7. Limit cheese intake, ice cream, sour cream, and imitation cream products. Most dairy products contain a high fat content.
9. Eat beans, rice, pasta, potatoes, whole grain cereals, vegetables, and fruits; if you are a man, eat what you want within reason. If you are a woman, eat these complex carbohydrates in moderation. (See the Unlimited Vegetable list on page 90.)

10. Eat no pies, cakes, cookies, or candies except on your pig-out meal (described in Chapter Ten).
11. Allow yourself one pig-out meal per week. Mark your calendar in advance for the day you choose to take it.

To get rid of the fat on your body, you first must get rid of the fat in your diet. In all my years in medical practice and research, I have yet to see a case of fat deficiency.

If you have not thought about fat in food before, I want to make you self-conscious about it now. You must start learning which foods contain the most fat. You will want to avoid these foods. To get you started creating your own set of rules, I'm giving you a list that I share with my patients.

Fat-Eating Rules

1. All red meat contains a large amount of fat. Eat it only on special occasions. Incidentally, my father was a beef producer. Can you imagine the reception I get when I visit my parents' home?
2. For your meat dishes, use only chicken or fish. Take the skin off the chicken before eating it.
3. In general, avoid all preprepared baked foods, especially dessert varieties. Most food manufacturers have used cheap fats such as lard and coconut oil. Over 35 to 40 percent of the calories in these foods come from fat. I could hardly bring myself to list coconuts in the Fat Awareness Table. They have so much saturated fat that it gives me a heart attack trying to write about it. Seven of this country's major cereal and bread manufacturers, including General Mills, Pillsbury, Borden, Ralston Purina, Keebler, and Pepperidge Farm, announced that they no longer use palm or coconut oil in the manufacturing process. Other food manufacturers are working to eliminate the use of coconut and palm oils. Consumers demanded it.
4. Avoid nuts in general if you're trying to lose weight.

Even though I feel most nuts are nutritionally sound foods to include in your diet, this does not hold true if you are trying to lose weight. Think about it. Which is more filling? Ten Spanish peanuts or an orange?

5. Fast food restaurants are okay if you don't step up to the main counter, and instead stumble to the salad bar.

6. Junk foods, in general—chips, pizzas, hot dogs, and similar foods—do not fit into the Ultrafit State. Work on your self-discipline to avoid potato chips and tortilla chips. Candy lovers must realize that over 60 percent of the calories in a chocolate bar come from fat. Chocolate candy has no place in a reducing diet. Regular ice cream contains over 65 percent fat. Try low-fat frozen yogurt, an elegant dessert that tastes much the same as ice cream.

Notice that I did not discuss saturated versus unsaturated fat in your diet. I feel that *all excess fat has no place in your diet* if you take long-term weight control and reaching the Ultrafit State seriously.

Fat/Protein/Carbohydrate

The Ultrafit Maintenance Diet contains the ideal percentages of fat, protein, and carbohydrate for women and men.

Let me repeat. Women should eat:

10 percent dietary calories from fat

15 to 20 percent dietary calories from protein

70 to 75 percent dietary calories from carbohydrate.

Men should eat:

10 percent dietary calories from fat

10 to 15 percent dietary calories from protein

75 to 80 percent dietary calories from carbohydrate.

Why do I recommend that women eat 5 percent more of their total calorie intake as protein than men? Remember, a woman consumes, in general, fewer calories than a man.

If she ate the same percentages as a man, she would lose muscle mass. Her muscle mass loss would deplete her mitochondria and force her to eat even fewer calories to avoid gaining weight. Remember, without the mitochondria you don't burn calories as efficiently. You store extra calories as fat.

Here's another simple rule of thumb you can follow if you are a woman. Never eat more than 17 grams of fat a day. By following this simple rule, your percentages of 10/15 to 20/70 to 75 will follow.

If you are a man, never eat more than 31 grams of fat a day.

Your Diet

Follow the Ultrafit Commandments. If you follow the Commandments, you do not need to worry about your 10/15 to 20/70 to 75 percentages for a woman, and the 10/10 to 15/75 to 80 percentages for a man.

To help you get started in your menu planning, I created one week's menus for the 1500- and for the 2500-calorie Ultrafit Maintenance Diets. Notice that I listed the grams of fat/protein/carbohydrate for each day's meals. This should give you an idea of an Ultrafit Maintenance Diet meal for a day.

Let me show you how I used the Ultrafit Maintenance Diet principles to teach Marge, a homemaker and one of my patients, how to prepare her food and plan her menus. She, like Art, weighed her ideal weight. She carried her 140 pounds on her five-foot, eight-inch frame with a certain grace. Yet, when we performed a serum blood cholesterol, we found that she had an elevated level, 270 milligrams percent. When I measured her percent body fat with skin calipers, I discovered her percent body fat was too high.

"Tell me, Marge," I said, "tell me what you eat and how

you prepare your foods." She ate sparingly. For breakfast she usually had a slice of whole wheat toast with a small sausage patty, sometimes with a strip of bacon, or a slice of cheddar cheese melted on the toast.

At lunch, she prepared a sandwich using thinly sliced whole wheat bread and bologna. Marge rarely ate out at lunch, so she generally ate the same foods, bologna sandwiches spread with one of her many varieties of mustards. Sometimes she substituted grilled sausages for the bologna.

Because her husband enjoyed pot roast and other beef dishes, she served a roast or steak at least twice a week. Over a period of ten years, these small servings of food filled with fat—beef, sausages, bacon, bologna, cheddar cheese—accumulated as fat on Marge's body and increased her cholesterol level.

And so began Marge's education in cooking and menu planning to lower the fat on her body by lowering the fat in her food. I encouraged her to use the mustards she loved. They contain little or no fat. I suggested that she begin using chicken, with the skin removed, and fish as her main courses. Instead of using butter, sour cream, or olive oil to flavor and cook her foods, I suggested that she begin cooking with herbs and use a nonstick cooking spray instead of fat.

"Have you ever tried," I asked her, "eating low-fat cottage cheese or yogurt for breakfast instead of those meats and fatty cheeses?" Marge began to catch on. "What about sliced turkey for lunch?" she asked.

"Yes," I encouraged her, "and because you love to cook, why not bake a batch of your favorite oatmeal cookies and eat two of those for dessert instead of that ice cream? Or try this bran muffin recipe and eat a large bran muffin for breakfast. You don't need to eat meat or concentrated protein with every meal.

"Think about your husband's health, too. Try to wean him from eating so much beef. He can eat the same foods you eat, only in larger quantities."

I discussed the menus with her, pointing out that the only

difference between her 1500-calorie Ultrafit Maintenance Diet and his 2500-calorie Maintenance Diet came in the quantities.

You must study these menus to make the same discovery.

I shared with Marge most of the recipes you will find in Chapter Eight, "The Ultrafit Diet Cookbook." In addition, I suggested that she secure a copy of Jane Brody's book *Good Food*. It contains superb low-fat recipes. "Use the *American Heart Association Cookbook*. Pick up a copy of the Pritikin cookbook, too," I said.

In planning your one week' menus for the 1500-calorie and 2500-calorie Ultrafit Diets, I've primarily used the Calorie/Fat/Protein/Carbohydrates/Content of Commonly Used Foods Table to calculate the grams of fat, protein, and carbohydrate. You may notice that gram figures vary from sourcebook to sourcebook. Do not worry. I want you to be flexible. In fact, I did not calculate the grams of fat and protein for the menus' fruits and vegetables because they provide only small amounts of fat and protein. You'll find the starred recipes in the menus in Chapter Eight, "The Ultrafit Diet Cookbook." Each menu item equals one serving of a recipe unless I tell you to add more or less.

Sample Menus

1500 Calories

DAY ONE

BREAKFAST	½ grapefruit *Hot Oatmeal, served with 1 teaspoon brown sugar 1 medium banana beverage of your choice
LUNCH	½ cup low-fat cottage cheese, sprinkled with chopped chives and parsley *2 slices whole wheat toast

1 medium orange
6 dates
beverage of your choice

SNACK   1 medium apple

DINNER   *Coq au Vin, served with 1 carrot, 1 large
potato
*1 Buttermilk Roll
tossed salad, seasoned with *Vinaigrette
Dressing
*Banana "Ice Cream"
beverage of your choice

1399 calories   59 gm protein   11 gm fat   239 gm carbohydrate

---

DAY TWO

BREAKFAST   ½ cantaloupe
*Herb-Scrambled Egg
*1 Bran Muffin
beverage of your choice

LUNCH   *Vegetable-Poached Chicken Breast, served
as sandwich with *2 slices
whole wheat bread
lettuce leaves and tomato slice, seasoned
with *Vinaigrette Dressing
3 dried apricot halves
beverage of your choice

SNACK   1 medium pear

DINNER   *Shrimp Creole, served with ⅔ cup steamed
white rice
tossed salad, seasoned with *Vinaigrette
Dressing
*Fruit Salad

3 ounces wine or apple juice
⅓ cup raisins

1520 calories   70 gm protein   19 gm fat   215 gm carbohydrate

---

DAY THREE

BREAKFAST
½ grapefruit
1½ servings *Hot Oatmeal, served with ½ cup skim milk
1 teaspoon brown sugar   ⅓ cup raisins
beverage of your choice

LUNCH
*1 toasted Bagel, served with 1 ounce slice Monterey Jack cheese
lettuce leaves and sliced tomato, seasoned with *Vinaigrette Dressing
1 medium banana
beverage of your choice

SNACK
1 medium apple
6 dates

DINNER
*Chicken with Pasta
tossed salad, seasoned with *Cilantro Dressing
3 ounces red wine or apple juice
1 cup white or red grapes
beverage of your choice

1519 calories   42 gm protein   13.5 gm fat   245 gm carbohydrate

---

DAY FOUR

BREAKFAST
½ cantaloupe
*Spring Omelet
*1 Applesauce Muffin
beverage of your choice

LUNCH   1 medium baked potato, stuffed with ¼ cup
                     low-fat cottage cheese with chopped chives
                     steamed broccoli, seasoned with *Vinai-
                     grette Dressing
                     1 medium banana
                     6 dates
                     beverage of your choice

SNACK   1 medium apple
                     ⅓ cup raisins

DINNER   *Mexican Chicken, served with 1 cup
                     steamed white rice
                     tossed salad, seasoned with *Cilantro
                     Dressing
                     *Fluffy Lime Pudding
                     1 medium orange
                     beverage of your choice

1490 calories   53 gm protein   16 gm fat   276 gm carbohydrate

DAY FIVE

BREAKFAST   1 medium banana
                     ¾ cup (1½ ounces) bran fiber cereal
                     ½ cup skim milk
                     beverage of your choice

LUNCH   *Tuna Salad, served as sandwich with
                     *2 slices whole wheat bread
                     lettuce leaves   sliced tomato
                     1 medium apple
                     beverage of your choice

SNACK   ⅓ cup raisins

DINNER   *Chicken-Mushroom Cutlet
                     1 cup steamed parsley potatoes

steamed green beans, seasoned with *Herb
Dressing
*1 Buttermilk Roll
1 cup fresh diced pineapple
beverage of your choice

1475 calories   63 gm protein   16 gm fat   260 gm carbohydrate

---

DAY SIX

BREAKFAST ½ grapefruit
*Parsley-Poached Egg
*1 Applesauce Muffin
beverage of your choice

LUNCH 1 medium pear, cut in half, served with
½ cup low-fat cottage cheese with chives
*1 toasted Bagel
6 dates
beverage of your choice

SNACK 1 medium banana

DINNER *3 Chicken Enchiladas
2 corn tortillas
tossed salad, seasoned with *Cilantro
Dressing
*Peach Crisp
beverage of your choice

1481 calories   59 gm protein   18 gm fat   238 gm carbohydrate

---

DAY SEVEN

BREAKFAST 1 medium peach
½ cup low-fat vanilla yogurt
*2 slices whole wheat toast
beverage of your choice

LUNCH	*Herb-Poached Chicken Breast, served as sandwich with *2 slices whole wheat bread lettuce leaves sliced tomato 1 medium banana
SNACK	1 medium apple
DINNER	*1½ cups Seasoned Pinto Beans *2 pieces Corn Bread steamed yellow squash, seasoned with *1 tablespoon Corn Relish 1 medium tangerine *Banana "Ice Cream" beverage of your choice

1530 calories   58 gm protein   19 gm fat   262 gm carbohydrate

2500 Calories

DAY ONE

BREAKFAST	½ grapefruit *1½ servings Hot Oatmeal, served with 2 teaspoons brown sugar ½ cup skim milk *2 toasted Bagels beverage of your choice
LUNCH	1 cup low-fat cottage cheese, sprinkled with chopped chives and parsley *3 slices whole wheat toast 1 medium orange 10 dates beverage of your choice
SNACK	1 medium banana *1 Bagel

DINNER   *Coq au Vin, served with 1½ carrots, 1 large
                potato
               *2 Buttermilk Rolls
               tossed salad, seasoned with *Vinaigrette
               Dressing
               *Banana "Ice Cream"
               beverage of your choice

SNACK   6 dried apricots

2499 calories   79 gm protein   25 gm fat   486 gm carbohydrate

DAY TWO

BREAKFAST ½ cantaloupe
               *Herb-Scrambled Egg
               *2 Bran Muffins
               beverage of your choice

SNACK   1 medium banana

LUNCH   *Vegetable-Poached Chicken Breast, served
               as sandwich with *2 slices
               whole wheat bread
               lettuce leaves   sliced tomato seasoned with
               *Vinaigrette Dressing
               1 medium banana
               beverage of your choice

SNACK   1 medium pear
               ⅔ cup raisins

DINNER   *Shrimp Creole, served with 1½ cups
               steamed white rice
               tossed salad, seasoned with *Vinaigrette
               Dressing
               *Fruit Salad
               3 ounces wine or apple juice

SNACK   1 medium banana
                  *1 Bran Muffin

2493 calories   66 gm protein   22 gm fat   503 gm carbohydrate

---

DAY THREE

BREAKFAST   1 medium banana   ⅓ cup raisins
                  *1½ servings Hot Oatmeal served with 2 tea-
                  spoons brown sugar
                  ½ cup skim milk
                  *1 slice Jelly Roll
                  beverage of your choice

LUNCH   *2 toasted Bagels, served with 1 ounce slice
                  Monterey Jack cheese
                  lettuce leaves and sliced tomato, seasoned
                  with *Vinaigrette Dressing
                  1 medium banana
                  1 medium orange
                  beverage of your choice

SNACK   1 medium apple
                  6 dates

DINNER   *Chicken with Pasta
                  tossed salad, seasoned with *Cilantro
                  Dressing
                  3 ounces red wine or apple juice
                  1 cup white or red grapes
                  beverage of your choice

SNACK   1 medium banana
                  ½ cup raisins

2466 calories   65 gm protein   17 gm fat   428 gm carbohydrate

DAY FOUR

BREAKFAST	½ cantaloupe *2 servings Spring Omelet *2 Applesauce Muffins 1 cup white or red grapes beverage of your choice
LUNCH	1 large baked potato, stuffed with ¼ cup low-fat cottage cheese with chopped chives steamed broccoli, seasoned with *Vinaigrette Dressing 1 medium banana 6 dates beverage of your choice
SNACK	1 medium apple ⅔ cup raisins
DINNER	*Mexican Chicken, served with 1 cup steamed white rice 2 hot corn tortillas tossed salad, seasoned with *Cilantro Dressing *Fluffy Lime Pudding 1 medium orange beverage of your choice
SNACK	1 medium pear

2506 calories   66 gm protein   26 gm fat   473 gm carbohydrate

DAY FIVE

BREAKFAST	1 medium banana ¾ cup (1½ ounces) bran fiber cereal ½ cup skim milk

pear
beverage of your choice

LUNCH   *Tuna Salad, served as 2 sandwiches with
*4 slices whole wheat bread
lettuce leaves   sliced tomato
1 medium apple (½ can be diced and added
to sandwich)
½ cup raisins (¼ cup can be added to
sandwich)
beverage of your choice

SNACK   1 medium orange
*1 Bagel

DINNER   *Chicken-Mushroom Cutlet
1 cup steamed parsley potatoes
steamed fresh green beans, seasoned with
*Herb Dressing
*2 Buttermilk Rolls
1 cup diced fresh pineapple

SNACK   1 medium banana
6 dates

2482 calories   81 gm protein   17 gm fat   465 gm carbohydrate

DAY SIX

BREAKFAST   1 medium banana
*2 servings Parsley-Poached Eggs
*3 Applesauce Muffins
beverage of your choice

LUNCH   1½ fresh pears, cut in half, served with
1 cup low-fat cottage cheese, with chives
*1 toasted Bagel
beverage of your choice

SNACK   1 medium banana
                6 dates

DINNER   *4 Chicken Enchiladas
                4 corn tortillas
                tossed salad, seasoned with *Cilantro
                Dressing
                *Peach Crisp
                beverage of your choice

2495 calories   79 gm protein   27 gm fat   413 gm carbohydrate

---

DAY SEVEN

BREAKFAST   1 medium banana
                ⅓ cup (1½ ounces) GrapeNuts
                ½ cup skim milk
                *3 slices whole wheat toast
                1 medium peach
                beverage of your choice

LUNCH   *Herb-Poached Chicken Breast, served as 2
                sandwiches with
                *4 slices whole wheat bread
                lettuce leaves   sliced tomato
                10 dates
                beverage of your choice

SNACK   1 medium apple
                *1 Bagel

DINNER   *1½ cups Seasoned Pinto Beans
                *2 pieces Corn Bread
                steamed yellow squash, seasoned with
                *½ cup Corn Relish
                tossed salad, seasoned with *Vinaigrette
                Dressing

*Banana "Ice Cream"
beverage of your choice

SNACK   1 medium pear
6 prunes

2497 calories · 86 gm protein · 28 gm fat · 427 gm carbohydrate

FAT AWARENESS TABLE

	PORTION	FAT CONTENT	TOTAL CALORIES PER SERVING
Fat Products			
Oils: corn, olive, peanut, palm, safflower, sesame	1 tbs.	14 grams	120
Butter, lard	1 tbs.	14 grams	120
Mayonnaise, regular	1 tbs.	11 grams	101
Mayonnaise, light	1 tbs.	4 grams	45
Nonstick cooking spray	2 seconds	0.8 grams	8
Dairy Products			
Skim Milk	1 cup	trace	90
½% Milk	1 cup	1 gram	95
2% Milk	1 cup	5 grams	120
½% Buttermilk	1 cup	1 gram	100
3.8% Whole Milk	1 cup	9 grams	160
Condensed Milk	1 cup	27 grams	982
Sour Cream	2 tbs.	4 grams	25
Half & Half Cream	2 tbs.	4 grams	40
Whipping Cream	2 tbs.	11 grams	110
Ice Cream	1 cup	14 grams	257
Nonfat Yogurt	1 cup	0.8 grams	120
Fruited Yogurt	1 cup	3 grams	230
Cheeses			
American, Blue	1 oz.	9 grams	105
Mozzarella & Monterey Jack	1 oz.	4.5 grams	72

Feta	1 oz.	5.5 grams	86
Parmesan	1 oz.	9.6 grams	119
Neufchatel	1 oz.	7 grams	75
Ricotta, skim milk	1 oz.	2 grams	43
Cream Cheese	1 oz.	10 grams	99
Gouda	1 oz.	8 grams	100
Brie	1 oz.	8 grams	98
Swiss, Cheddar, Brick, Colby	1 oz.	9.5 grams	115
Cottage Cheese (regular)	½ cup	8 grams	135
Cottage Cheese (Low-fat)	½ cup	4 grams	100

Lunch Meats

Turkey Ham	1 oz.	1.5 grams	35
Boiled Ham	1 oz.	5.5 grams	70
Salami	1 oz.	6 grams	75
Frank—Chicken	1 oz.	8 grams	85
Frank—Meat	1 oz.	8 grams	90
Bologna	1 oz.	8 grams	90
Liverwurst	1 oz.	9 grams	139

Notice that lunch meats make poor choices in your diet. You need to get rid of them. Hot dogs made only of cereal belong in your diet. They don't sell that kind at ballgames. Now you see why I recommend you use water-packed tuna and skinless chicken breast for sandwiches.

Fish

Haddock	3.5 oz.	0.1 grams	80
Cod	3.5 oz.	0.3 grams	80
Sole	3.5 oz.	0.4 grams	68
Flounder	3.5 oz.	0.4 grams	70
Red Snapper	3.5 oz.	0.8 grams	90
Halibut	3.5 oz.	1.2 grams	100
Perch	3.5 oz.	1.5 grams	95
Brook Trout	3.5 oz.	2.1 grams	100
Swordfish	3.5 oz.	4 grams	120
Mackerel—Pacific	3.5 oz.	7.5 grams	165
Mackerel—Atlantic	3.5 oz.	12.5 grams	195

Chinook Salmon	3.5 oz.	15 grams	225
Tuna—Water Pack	3 oz.	0.6 grams	120
Tuna—Oil Pack	3 oz.	8.5 grams	200
Pink Salmon— Canned	3 oz.	6 grams	150
Silver Salmon— Canned	3 oz.	8.2 grams	160

Meat—Fat Trimmed

Chicken	3 oz.	3 grams	110
Beef—Round Steak	3 oz.	4.5 grams	190
Sirloin Steak	3 oz.	7 grams	180
Flank Steak	3 oz.	7.5 grams	200
Ground Beef— Lean	3 oz.	10 grams	210
Lamb	3 oz.	7 grams	170
Liver, Calf	3 oz.	11 grams	222
Ground Turkey	3 oz.	11.2 grams	150
Pot Roast—Lean	3 oz.	12 grams	230
Pork Chop	3 oz.	22 grams	301

Legumes

Lentils	1 cup cooked	0.1 grams	200
Peas—Split	1 cup cooked	0.5 grams	230
Beans—Navy, Kidney, Pinto	1 cup cooked	1 gram	225

Eggs

Whole Egg	1 medium	6 grams	80
Egg White	1	trace	15

Nuts and Seeds

Cashews	1 oz. (12–14 nuts)	13 grams	150
Sunflower Seeds	1 oz.	13 grams	150
Peanuts—Raw	1 oz.	14 grams	170
Walnuts	1 oz.	14 grams	170
Pistachios	1 oz.	16 grams	180
Almonds	1 oz.	16 grams	180
Filberts	1 oz.	19 grams	190

| Pecans | 1 oz. | 22 | grams | 215 |
| Macadamia Nuts | 1 oz. | 24 | grams | 230 |

Other High-Fat Foods

Avocado	½	19	grams	188
Chocolate	1 oz.	15	grams	143
Coconut, grated	½ cup	14	grams	138

Nutritive Value of American Foods in Common Units, Agriculture Handbook No. 456. U.S. Department of Agriculture. Issued November 1975.

Becoming Ultrafit means that you commit yourself to changing your eating habits over time.

Life is not an exact science, it is an art.
—SAMUEL BUTLER

CHAPTER EIGHT

The Ultrafit Diet Cookbook

To assist you in getting acquainted with the Ultrafit way of cooking, I've supplied the recipes for dishes I've written into the 1000-, 1500-, and 2500-calorie menus. Each recipe gives the number of servings, and the number of calories and grams (g) of protein, fat, and carbohydrate per serving. In addition to the recipes used in the menus, I have supplied other recipes that can be used in place of dishes in the menus. I've written a note on these recipes, telling you which menu item you can replace with the recipe item. Of course, the daily nutritional counts of each recipe will vary slightly, but not enough to affect the diet you choose to follow.

The contents page for this cookbook section appears on p. xi.

Egg Dishes and Breakfast Cereals

Herb-Scrambled Egg

Serves 1

1 egg
1 tablespoon water

⅛ teaspoon of favorite fresh
herb (one-third the amount
if using dried herb)*

Beat egg slightly. Add water and fresh or dried herb. Beat
until all ingredients are incorporated. Spray skillet with nonstick cooking spray. Heat skillet over medium heat. When
hot, add egg. Lift and stir egg gently with wood spoon or
heatproof rubber scraper until set, about 3 minutes.

Per serving: 82 calories; 7 g protein; 5 g fat; 0 g carbohydrate

Parsley-Poached Egg

Serves 1

1 egg
1 cup water

1 parsley sprig, chopped

Add water to 1-quart saucepan, up to 2 inches. Bring water
to simmer (do not boil). Break egg into a shallow dish, tilt
dish, and slip egg into simmering water. Simmer egg 3 to 5
minutes, depending on your preference. Remove with slotted spoon. Sprinkle with freshly chopped parsley.

Per serving: 82 calories; 7 g protein; 5 g fat; 0 g carbohydrate

* See herb chart on pages 161–62.

Spring Omelet

Serves 1

1 egg
1 tablespoon water
½ small fresh tomato,
  chopped, divided

½ teaspoon chopped shallot,
  divided
¼ teaspoon chopped parsley

Beat water into egg. Spray small skillet with nonstick cooking spray. Heat pan over medium heat. When hot, add egg. Cook egg about 20 to 30 seconds, then tilt pan and with a nonstick spatula or fork, pull the edge of the omelet toward the center of the pan, allowing the still liquid egg to run beneath and cook. Continue around the omelet until egg is set.

Sprinkle egg with ⅔ of the tomato and shallot and all the parsley. Fold half of egg over ingredients and slide onto serving plate. Sprinkle with remaining tomato and shallot.

Per serving: 82 calories; 7 g protein; 5 g fat; 0 g carbohydrate

Hot Oatmeal

Serves 1

1 ounce (approximately ⅓ cup)
  uncooked oatmeal

⅔ cup water

Bring water to rolling boil. Add oats and cook 5 minutes, stirring occasionally. Cover, remove from heat and serve in 2 to 3 minutes.

Per serving: 100 calories; 5 g protein; 2 g fat; 18 g carbohydrate

Hot Cream of Wheat

Serves 1

1 ounce (2½ tablespoons) un-   1½ cups water
cooked Cream of Wheat

Bring water to rolling boil. Add cereal, stirring constantly.
Bring to boil again. Reduce heat and cook for 10 minutes,
stirring constantly.

Per serving: 100 calories; 3 g protein; 0 g fat; 22 g carbohydrate

Beverages

Each day you should drink at least 8 cups of water. In
addition to water, other Ultrafit Diet beverages of choice
include those served without cream and sugar. Drink teas
of all kinds: herb, lemon, iced or hot. Restrict your coffee
to two cups per day to avoid excess caffeine. Calorie-free,
caffeine-free soft drinks and ices belong, if you enjoy them.

Breads

One serving of bread from any one of the following recipes
can be used in any menu in which I call for one bread serving.
In addition, you can use 1 corn, flour, whole wheat, or oat
bran tortilla, or 1 whole wheat pocket bread as one serving
of bread.

Buttermilk Rolls

Makes 24 rolls

2 packages dry yeast
¼ cup warm water
¼ cup sugar, divided
5 cups all-purpose flour,
  divided
1 teaspoon salt

½ teaspoon soda
1½ cups lowfat buttermilk,
  heated until warm to the
  touch
½ cup safflower oil

Combine yeast, water, and 1 tablespoon of sugar in a small bowl and stir. In a large bowl, combine remaining sugar, 4 cups of flour, salt, and soda.

Stir liquid mixture from small bowl, warm buttermilk, and oil into large bowl of dry ingredients. Mix well. Stir in remaining flour to make a stiff dough.

Let rest 10 minutes, then knead for 5 minutes. Pinch off 24 pieces of dough, roll, forming into balls, and place on a baking sheet sprayed with nonstick cooking spray.

Cover with light towel and let rise 30 minutes. Bake in a 400° oven for 8 to 10 minutes.

Per roll: 140 calories; 3 g protein, 5 g fat; 21 g carbohydrate

Bran Muffins

Makes 12 muffins

1 cup all-purpose flour
⅓ cup brown sugar
½ teaspoon baking soda
1¼ cups 100% bran cereal
2½ teaspoons baking powder

½ teaspoon salt
1 egg
3 tablespoons safflower oil
1 cup skim milk

Combine flour, brown sugar, baking soda, bran cereal, baking powder, and salt, and mix well. Stir in egg, oil, and milk until dry ingredients are just moistened. Spray muffin tins with nonstick cooking spray and fill ¾ full. Bake in a 400° oven for 15 to 20 minutes.

Per muffin: 106 calories; 3 g protein; 2 g fat; 16 g carbohydrate

Applesauce Muffins

Makes 12 muffins

2 cups all-purpose flour	1 egg
2½ teaspoons baking powder	¼ cup honey
½ teaspoon baking soda	¾ cup raisins
1 teaspoon cinnamon	
1⅓ cups unsweetened applesauce	

Combine flour, baking powder, baking soda, and cinnamon in a large bowl. To dry ingredients, add applesauce, egg, and honey. Stir mixture until just moistened. Stir in raisins. Spray muffin tin with nonstick cooking spray and fill ¾ full. Bake in a 375° oven for 20 minutes.

Per muffin: 161 calories; 3 g protein; 2 g fat; 30 g carbohydrate

Whole Wheat Muffins

Makes 12 muffins

1 cup whole wheat flour	1 cup skim milk
1 cup all-purpose flour	2 egg whites
2½ teaspoons baking powder	¼ cup safflower oil
½ teaspoon salt	½ cup raisins
¼ cup brown sugar	

Combine the flours, baking powder, salt, and sugar in a large bowl. Stir together the milk, egg whites, and oil. Add to the dry ingredients along with the raisins. Stir until just moistened. Spray muffin tin with nonstick cooking spray. Fill muffin cups until ¾ full. Bake in a 400° oven for 20 minutes.

Per muffin: 148 calories; 4 g protein; 5 g fat; 24 g carbohydrate

Bagels

Makes 12 bagels

2 packages dry yeast
2 cups whole wheat flour
4 tablespoons sugar, divided
2 teaspoons salt

1¾ cups very warm water
2 to 3 cups unbleached white flour

Combine the yeast, wheat flour, 3 tablespoons of sugar, and the salt in a mixing bowl. Add the water and stir well to dissolve the yeast. Stir in white flour, 1 cup at a time, to make a stiff dough.

Knead the dough on a floured board until smooth and satiny. Dough should be very firm. Cover with light cloth or plastic wrap and let rest for 20 minutes.

Divide dough into 12 portions. Shape into balls and poke your thumb through the center; pull to enlarge circles. Place on a baking sheet sprayed with nonstick cooking spray. Cover and let rise for 30 minutes.

Bring 3 quarts of water to a boil in a 5-quart pan. Add the remaining tablespoon of sugar. Lower the bagels into the water, 4 or 5 at a time, turning often for 5 minutes. Remove from the water with a slotted spoon and return to the baking sheet. Bake in a 375° oven for 30 minutes.

Per bagel: 148 calories; 4 g protein, 1 g fat; 32 g carbohydrate

Corn Bread

Makes 9 servings

1 cup yellow cornmeal	1 cup skim milk
1 cup all-purpose flour	1 egg
4 teaspoons baking powder	¼ cup corn oil
½ teaspoon salt	

Combine cornmeal, flour, baking powder, and salt. Add milk, egg, and corn oil. Beat until fairly smooth, about 1 minute. Spray 8-inch-square baking pan with nonstick cooking spray, add batter, and bake at 425° for 20 to 25 minutes.

Per serving: 176 calories; 5 g protein; 7 g fat; 23 g carbohydrate

Refrigerator Whole Wheat Bread

Makes 4 loaves (16 slices per loaf) or 2 loaves (32 slices per loaf)

3 cups skim milk	3 cups whole wheat flour
1 cup water	4½ tablespoons sugar
6 tablespoons corn oil	4 teaspoons salt
margarine	5 to 6 cups unbleached flour
2 packages dry yeast	

In a saucepan heat the milk, water, and margarine until warm to the touch and the margarine has melted. Pour mixture into a large bowl and stir in yeast. Let the mixture rest 5 minutes until yeast dissolves.

Add whole wheat flour, sugar, and salt and stir the batter for 2 minutes, or until well moistened. Stir in the unbleached flour a cup at a time until the dough is very stiff.

Turn out on a floured board and knead until the dough is smooth and elastic, adding flour as necessary. Cover the dough with a plastic wrap or light cloth and let rest 15 to 20 minutes.

Shape the dough into loaves and place in four 4 × 8-inch or two 5 × 9-inch pans sprayed with nonstick cooking spray. Cover with plastic wrap and refrigerate for 2 to 24 hours.

Remove from the refrigerator, unwrap, and let stand at room temperature for 10 minutes. Bake at 375° for 35 minutes.

Per slice: 67 calories; 2 g protein; 2 g fat; 11 g carbohydrate

Buttermilk Bran Bread

Makes 2 loaves, 32 slices per loaf

1 cup low-fat buttermilk
1 cup water
⅓ cup corn oil margarine
5 to 6 cups unbleached white flour, divided

1 package dry yeast
3 tablespoons sugar
½ cup unprocessed bran
2 teaspoons salt
¼ teaspoon baking powder

In a saucepan heat buttermilk, water, and margarine until warm to the touch, and the margarine melts.

Combine 2 cups of flour, the yeast, sugar, bran, salt, and baking powder in a large bowl. Add the liquids and beat well to dissolve the yeast. Add the remaining flour, one cup at a time, until the dough is very stiff.

Turn out onto a floured board and knead until the dough is smooth and elastic. Return to the bowl and cover with a light cloth or plastic wrap. Let rise in a warm place for 1 hour.

Punch down and shape into two loaves. Place in two 5 × 9-inch loaf pans sprayed with nonstick cooking spray, and let rise again for 1 hour. Bake in a 350° oven for 30 minutes.

Per slice: 82 calories; 3 g protein; 1 g fat; 15 g carbohydrate

Banana Bread

Makes 1 loaf, 12 slices

1½ cups all-purpose flour
½ cup sugar
2 teaspoons baking soda
½ teaspoon salt
½ cup bran cereal

3 ripe bananas, mashed
¼ cup low-fat buttermilk
3 tablespoons safflower oil
4 egg whites

Stir together flour, sugar, baking soda, salt, and bran cereal. Add bananas, buttermilk, oil, and egg whites. Stir until well blended. Pour into a 4 × 8-inch loaf pan sprayed with non-stick cooking spray. Bake in a 350° oven for 1 hour.

To microwave, cook on high power for 6 to 8 minutes and then brown in a 350° oven for 10 to 15 minutes.

Per slice: 126 calories; 4 g protein; 4 g fat; 21 g carbohydrate

Fruits

Worldwide marketing and efficient transportation allow you to buy fresh fruit throughout the year. The Ultrafit Diets use fruit in most meals. To help you determine the size serving of fruits in your Ultrafit Diet, I've created a list of fresh fruits that gives quantities equal to one serving. When in doubt about the size, remember that you want to eat a medium-size fruit or equivalent serving.

1 medium apple
3 medium apricots
1 medium banana
1 cup of berries: blackberries,
  blueberries, boysenberries,
  gooseberries, raspberries,
  strawberries

½ medium cantaloupe
10 cherries
2 medium figs
10 grapes, white or red
½ grapefruit
¹⁄₁₀ honeydew melon
1 medium mango
1 medium orange

1 medium peach
1 cup diced pineapple
2 medium plums

1 tangerine
1 cup watermelon pieces

Soups and Sandwiches

Chicken Soup with Rice
Serves 8

4 skinless, boneless chicken
  breast halves
8 carrots, peeled and diced
1 medium onion, diced
8 stalks celery, diced

3 sprigs parsley
8 cups water
Salt and pepper to taste
1 cup uncooked white rice
1 tablespoon chopped parsley

Add chicken breasts, carrots, onion, celery, and parsley to water and bring to a simmer. Cover and simmer 5 minutes. Remove chicken and parsley. Discard parsley. Add rice to vegetable soup and simmer 30 minutes. Dice chicken and stir into rice vegetable soup until chicken is heated through. Serve in bowls. Top each bowl of soup with chopped parsley.

Per serving: 224 calories; 15 g protein; 2 g fat; 33 g carbohydrate

Turkey-Vegetable Soup
Serves 8

2 turkey legs
2 quarts water
1 onion, chopped
8 carrots, peeled and diced
8 red potatoes, scrubbed and
  cubed

1 28-ounce can tomatoes, broken into pieces
2 packages frozen green beans
Salt and pepper to taste

Simmer the turkey legs in water until tender, about 1½ hours. Remove the legs from the broth and cool. Remove the meat from the bones. Discard the skin, bones, and tendons. Strain the broth and skim off all the fat. Return the broth and meat to the soup pot. Add all the vegetables except the green beans and return to simmer for 20 to 30 minutes. Add the green beans and continue simmering for an additional 15 to 20 minutes. Season with salt and pepper.

Per serving: 314 calories; 30 g protein; 6 g fat; 34 g carbohydrate

New England Seafood Chowder

Serves 6

2 medium potatoes, peeled and cubed
1 medium onion, diced
2 cups chicken broth, defatted
1 pound cod filets, cut into small pieces

1 6½-ounce can chopped clams, drained
2 cups skim milk
1 12-ounce can evaporated skim milk
Paprika

Cook potatoes and onion in broth until tender. Add fish and clams and simmer for 10 minutes. Stir in milks and simmer for 15 minutes longer, being careful not to boil. Serve in soup bowls garnished with a sprinkle of paprika.

Per serving: 181 calories; 21 g protein; 1 g fat; 22 g carbohydrate

Split Pea Soup

Serves 8

1 pound dried split peas
8 cups water
½ pound turkey ham cut into
   large pieces

1 medium onion, diced
2 tablespoons chopped cilantro
½ teaspoon black pepper
Salt to taste

Place split peas in water in a large soup pot. Bring to boil and boil for 2 minutes. Lower heat to simmer, add turkey ham, onion, and cilantro, and simmer, stirring occasionally, for 1½ to 2 hours. (Peas will lose their form and soup will thicken.) Add pepper and season with salt, depending on the saltiness of the turkey ham.

Per serving: 232 calories; 19 g protein; 2 g fat; 35 g carbohydrate

Vegetable-Poached Chicken Breast

Serves 1

Water
1 small carrot, diced
1 small white onion, diced
1 small celery stick, diced

1 skinless, boneless chicken
   breast half
Dash of freshly ground black
   pepper

Add up to 3 inches of water in a 1-quart saucepan. Add vegetables and pepper. Bring to a simmer. Add chicken breast, cover pan, and simmer 5 minutes. Remove breast, cool, and slice for sandwich preparation.

Per serving: 160 calories; 26 g protein; 5 g fat; 1 g carbohydrate

Herb-Poached Chicken Breast
Serves 1

Water
1 parsley sprig
1 small bay leaf
1 small white onion, diced

1 sprig fresh thyme, or ½ teaspoon dried
1 skinless, boneless chicken
 breast half

Add up to 3 inches of water in a 1-quart saucepan. Add
parsley, bay leaf, onion, and thyme. Bring to a simmer. Add
chicken breast, cover pan, and simmer 5 minutes. Remove
breast, cool, and slice for sandwich preparation.

Per serving: 160 calories; 26 g protein; 5 g fat; 1 g carbohydrate

Turkey Burgers
Serves 8

1 pound ground turkey   Salt and pepper to taste

Divide ground meat into 8 equal portions and shape into
burger patties. Spray skillet with nonstick cooking spray.
Heat skillet and sauté burgers.

Per serving: 108 calories; 18 g protein; 8 g fat; 0 g carbohydrate

Main Dishes

Coq au Vin

Serves 4

4 skinless, boneless chicken
 breast halves
½ teaspoon dried thyme
4 to 6 carrots, peeled and left
 whole
¼ teaspoon salt

4 medium white potatoes,
 peeled and cut in half
½ cup dry red wine
1 teaspoon cornstarch
½ cup cold water

Brown chicken breasts in dutch oven sprayed with nonsticking cooking spray. Add thyme, carrots, salt, potatoes, and red wine. Cover and simmer for 45 minutes. Add more water if necessary. Mix cornstarch with cold water. Add, stirring constantly, to simmering sauce to thicken.

Per serving: 346 calories; 42 g protein; 3 g fat; 45 g carbohydrate

Chicken and Pasta

Serves 4

4 skinless, boneless chicken
 breast halves
¼ white onion, peeled and
 chopped
1 16-ounce can tomato sauce

1 teaspoon dried basil
1 teaspoon dried oregano
8 ounces dried pasta (spinach,
 noodles, shells, or rotini),
 cooked

Cut chicken breasts into small cubes. Brown chicken and onion in saucepan sprayed with nonstick cooking spray. Add tomato sauce, basil, and oregano. Simmer until tender, about 15 minutes. Serve over pasta.

Per serving: 328 calories; 23 g protein; 2 g fat; 52 g carbohydrate

Mexican Chicken

Serves 4

4 skinless, boneless chicken
  breast halves
¼ white onion, peeled and
  chopped

1 teaspoon chili powder
½ teaspoon cumin
1 8-ounce can salt-free tomato
  sauce

Brown chicken and onion in dutch oven sprayed with non-stick cooking spray. Combine chili powder and cumin and add to tomato sauce. Pour over chicken and simmer, covered, for 15 minutes, or until chicken is tender.

Per serving: 179 calories; 28 g protein; 3 g fat; 6 g carbohydrate

Chicken-Mushroom Cutlet

Serves 1

1 skinless, boneless chicken
  breast half

⅛ teaspoon dried rosemary
½ cup mushrooms, sliced

Place chicken breast between sheets of wax paper and pound with mallet until flattened to about ⅜ inch. Rub chicken with dried rosemary. Spray a skillet with nonstick cooking spray, heat skillet, and add chicken breast and mushrooms. Sauté chicken about 3 minutes per side. Serve immediately.

Per serving: 160 calories; 28 g protein; 3 g fat; 1 g carbohydrate

Chicken Enchiladas

Makes 4 enchiladas

1½ cups water, divided
1 skinless, boneless chicken
   breast half
1 teaspoon chili powder
½ teaspoon cumin
4 ounces salt-free tomato sauce

4 corn tortillas
¼ ounce grated Monterey Jack
   cheese
1 medium white onion, peeled
   and finely chopped

Bring 1 cup water to boil in 1-quart saucepan, add chicken, cover and simmer about 5 minutes. Remove chicken, discard water, cool meat, and shred or finely chop.

Mix chili powder and cumin in the saucepan with tomato sauce and ½ cup water. Simmer until the sauce thickens slightly, about 10 minutes.

Place tortillas in a loosely closed plastic bag and warm in the microwave until limp. (These may be warmed in an oven by wrapping the tortillas in a damp cloth and then in foil.)

Spray 8 × 8-inch baking dish with nonstick cooking spray. With tongs, dip warmed tortillas one by one in the hot tomato sauce mixture, then lay them flat in the baking dish. Sprinkle ¼ of the chicken and ¼ of the cheese across the middle of the tortilla. Then roll the tortilla and place it seam-side down in the baking dish.

After making the 4 enchiladas, pour the remaining sauce over the enchiladas in the baking dish. Garnish with finely chopped onions and bake in a 350° oven for 10 to 15 minutes.

Per enchilada: 111 calories; 6 g protein; 3 g fat; 11 g carbohydrate

Stir-Fried Chicken

Serves 4

2 skinless, boneless chicken
   breast halves, thinly sliced
2 scallions, cut into bite-size
   pieces
3 celery stalks, cut on the
   diagonal
1 green bell pepper, diced

1 bunch fresh broccoli, cut into
   bite-size pieces
4 cups fresh bean sprouts
1 teaspoon cornstarch dissolved
   in ½ cup cold water
Salt to taste

Spray nonstick cooking spray on bottom of a large skillet or
wok and heat until medium-hot. Stir-fry chicken and scallions until chicken loses its pink color. Add celery, green
pepper, broccoli, and bean sprouts; stir-fry about 1 minute,
cover, and steam about 3 minutes. Add cornstarch mixture
and stir until thickened. Add salt to taste. Serve with hot
rice, using the amount stated in the menu.

Per serving: 108 calories; 17 g protein; 2 g fat; 7 g carbohydrate

Baked Chicken Breasts with
Corn Bread Dressing

Serves 6

1 pan corn bread, cooked and
   crumbled (see recipe on page
   134)
1 medium white onion,
   chopped
6 celery stalks, chopped

⅛ teaspoon black pepper
1 teaspoon dried sage
¾ cup defatted chicken broth
6 skinless, boneless chicken
   breast halves
1 teaspoon dried tarragon

Crumble corn bread in a large bowl. Stir in onion, celery,
pepper, sage, and chicken broth. Spray a large baking/serv-
ing dish with nonstick cooking spray. Pour corn bread mix-

ture into dish and pack down. Rub chicken breasts with tarragon and place chicken on top of dressing and bake in a 350° oven for 1 hour.

Per serving: 270 calories; 30 g protein; 5 g fat; 22 g carbohydrate

Turkey Spaghetti

Serves 4

½ pound ground turkey
½ medium white onion, chopped
1 16-ounce can salt-free tomato sauce

½ teaspoon dried oregano
½ teaspoon dried basil
½ cup water
8 ounces spaghetti or vermicelli, cooked

Spray skillet with nonstick cooking spray. Heat pan to medium hot and brown turkey and onion. Add tomato sauce, oregano, basil, and water. Simmer, covered, for about 30 minutes. Serve over hot pasta.

Per serving: 356 calories; 18 g protein; 8 g fat; 51 g carbohydrate

Soft Turkey Tacos

Makes 16 tacos

1 pound ground turkey
2 tablespoons finely chopped white onion
1 teaspoon chili powder
1 teaspoon ground cumin

¼ cup water
16 corn tortillas
½ head lettuce, shredded
4 medium tomatoes, chopped

Spray skillet with nonstick cooking spray and heat. Brown turkey and onions. Add chili powder, cumin, and water. Cover and simmer for 15 to 20 minutes. Warm tortillas in plastic in microwave or wrapped in foil in the oven. To serve, place 2 tablespoons turkey filling in warmed tortilla, top with lettuce and tomato, roll tortilla around filling and eat with your fingers.

Per taco: 107 calories; 6 g protein; 4 g fat; 10 g carbohydrate

Shrimp Creole

Serves 4

3 to 4 celery stalks, chopped
¼ white onion, peeled and chopped
1 green bell pepper, seeded and diced
1 16-ounce can tomatoes, broken

1 8-ounce can tomato sauce
1 pound peeled, deveined shrimp
⅛ cup mild picante sauce

Spray the bottom of dutch oven with nonstick cooking spray. Add celery, onion, and green pepper and cook until onion is translucent. Add tomatoes and tomato sauce; cover and simmer 15 to 20 minutes. Add shrimp and simmer until they turn pink and curl, about 6 minutes. Add picante sauce. Serve in bowls over rice, using the amount stated in menu.

Per serving: 244 calories; 39 g protein; 2 g fat; 17 g carbohydrate

Linguine with Clam Sauce

Serves 4

1 16-ounce can salt-free tomato sauce
½ teaspoon dried oregano
½ teaspoon dried basil

2 6½-ounce cans minced clams, drained
8 ounces linguine, cooked

Combine tomato sauce and herbs and simmer for 15 minutes. Add clams and simmer 10 more minutes. Serve over hot linguine.

Per serving: 291 calories; 16 g protein; 2 g fat; 50 g carbohydrate

Pan-Broiled Fish Filets

Serves 4

2 tablespoons all-purpose flour
2 tablespoons unprocessed
    wheat or oat bran
4 4-ounce filets of flounder,
    sole, or any nonoily fish

2 teaspoons corn oil margarine
Paprika
2 tablespoons finely chopped
    parsley
1 lemon, cut into wedges

Combine flour and bran and coat filets in mixture. Spray large iron skillet with nonstick cooking spray and heat skillet to medium hot. Melt margarine in skillet. Add filets and cook 3 to 5 minutes. Remove pan from heat and place under broiler, about 6 inches from heat, for 2 to 4 minutes until filets are golden. Sprinkle with paprika and parsley. Serve with lemon wedge.

Per serving: 123 calories; 16 g protein; 2 g fat; 5 g carbohydrate

Creoled Haddock

Serves 4

4 celery stalks, chopped
1 green bell pepper, diced
4 scallions, finely chopped
1 16-ounce can tomatoes, bro-
    ken into pieces

1½ teaspoons mild picante
    sauce
1 pound haddock or turbot
    filets

Combine celery, pepper, scallions, tomatoes, and picante sauce in saucepan, cover, and simmer for about 15 minutes. Place filets in a baking/serving dish and spread cooked vegetable mixture on top. Bake fish in a 400° oven for 5 to 10 minutes. Fish is done when it flakes easily.

Per serving: 120 calories; 18 g protein; 0 g fat; 6 g carbohydrate

Oriental Shrimp

Serves 4

2 scallions, diagonally sliced
2 cups diagonally sliced snow peas, ends and strings removed
1 cup diagonally sliced celery

1 cup sliced mushrooms
1 pound shrimp, shelled, deveined, and sliced lengthwise
1 teaspoon cornstarch dissolved in ¼ cup cold water

Coat large skillet or wok with nonstick cooking spray and heat to medium hot. Add scallions, snow peas, celery, and mushrooms and stir-fry for 3 to 5 minutes. Add the shrimp and continue to stir; cook until shrimp turn pink and curl. Add cornstarch mixture and stir until thickened. Serve over rice, using the amount stated in the menus.

Per serving: 153 calories; 22 g protein; 1 g fat; 15 g carbohydrate

Orange Roughy à l' Orange

Serves 4

4 4-ounce filets orange roughy (or any mild white fish)
¼ teaspoon salt
2 tablespoons orange juice

1 teaspoon grated orange rind
1 tablespoon safflower oil
Dash of nutmeg

Place filets in a baking dish coated with nonstick cooking spray. Combine salt, orange juice, orange rind, nutmeg, and oil. Pour over fish. Bake for 10 minutes in a 400° oven, until fish flakes.

Per serving: 133 calories; 18 g protein; 3 g fat; 4 g carbohydrate

Seasoned Pinto Beans

Serves 3

1 cup dry pinto beans, sorted and rinsed	1 medium onion, peeled and chopped
9 cups water (4 times)	3 dashes of hot sauce

To reduce the gas-forming tendency of beans, soak them in 9 cups of water for 4 to 5 hours. Discard the water. Add 9 cups of fresh water and cook for ½ hour. Discard the water. Add 9 cups of water and cook again and drain. Add 9 cups of water, onion, and hot sauce, and simmer for 4 hours. Check beans for doneness, and continue cooking until done.

Per serving: 221 calories; 14 g protein; 1 g fat; 40 g carbohydrate

Substitute Main-Dish Recipes

One serving of these recipes can be substituted for 1 main-dish serving in any of the dinner menus.

Baked Chicken with Barley

Serves 6

(1 serving can substitute for 1 main-dish serving
in any dinner menu)

1 cup chopped white onions	1 cup barley
½ cup chopped celery	3 cups defatted chicken broth
2 green bell peppers, seeded and chopped	6 skinless, boneless chicken breast halves
½ cup dry white wine	4 scallions, chopped
3 cups canned tomatoes, drained and broken into pieces	

Coat a large saucepan with nonstick cooking spray. Add the onion, celery, and green pepper and sauté for about 5 minutes. Add the wine, tomatoes, barley, and broth and bring to a boil. Reduce the heat, cover, and simmer for 30 minutes. Place vegetable-barley mixture in the bottom of a baking dish.

Coat a skillet with nonstick cooking spray, heat to medium hot, add chicken breasts, and brown about 2 minutes on each side. Place browned chicken breasts on top of vegetable-barley mixture. Cover and bake in a 350° oven for 20 minutes. Garnish with scallions.

Per serving: 337 calories; 33 g protein; 3 g fat; 40 g carbohydrate

Company Turkey Loaf

Serves 6

(1 serving can substitute for 1 main-dish serving
in any dinner menu)

1 cup finely chopped celery
½ cup finely chopped white
   onion
2 red bell peppers, seeded and
   diced
2 cups thinly sliced mushrooms, divided

½ teaspoon salt
½ teaspoon black pepper
1 cup fresh bread crumbs
½ cup chopped parsley
1 pound ground turkey

Coat a medium saucepan with nonstick cooking spray and
sauté the celery, onion, bell peppers, and 1 cup of mushrooms until slightly softened, about 5 minutes. Arrange remaining cup of mushroom slices on the bottom of a spray-
coated 5 × 9-inch loaf pan. Combine the sautéed vegetables,
salt, pepper, bread crumbs, and parsley with the turkey.
Place the mixture in the loaf pan and bake in a 375° oven
for 1 hour. Invert on a serving platter and allow to rest for
10 minutes before removing pan and slicing.

Per serving: 217 calories; 17 g protein; 11 g fat; 18 g carbohydrate

Flounder Florentine

Serves 4

(1 serving can substitute for 1 main-dish serving
in any dinner menu)

1 package frozen, chopped
   spinach
4 4-ounce flounder filets (or
   any mild white fish)
¼ cup chopped scallion

⅛ teaspoon paprika
½ teaspoon dried dill
¼ cup dry white wine
2 tablespoons lemon juice

Cook the spinach for 3 to 5 minutes or until thawed. Drain
well. Lay filets flat. Combine spinach and scallion and spread
a layer over each filet. Roll filets and fasten with toothpicks.
Place in a baking dish and sprinkle with paprika and dill.
Pour wine and lemon juice around the filets and bake in 350°
oven for 20 minutes, or until fish flakes. Serve with Dill-
Mustard Sauce (see recipe on page 166), if desired.

Per serving: 99 calories; 18 g protein; 1 g fat; 6 g carbohydrate

Seafood Pilaf

Serves 6

(1 serving can substitute for 1 main-dish serving
in any dinner menu)

1 cup thinly sliced scallion
1 large tomato, peeled, seeded,
   and chopped
½ cup minced parsley
½ cup dry white wine
1 6½-ounce can minced clams,
   drained and juice saved

2 cups water
1½ cups brown rice
½ pound bay scallops
½ pound shrimp, shelled and
   deveined

Coat a large saucepan with nonstick cooking spray and sauté
scallion. Add tomato and stir until softened, about 3 minutes.
Add parsley, wine, clam juice, water, and bring to a boil.
Stir in the rice, cover, and simmer for 30 minutes. Remove
covered pan from heat and let rest for 15 minutes. Uncover,
stir in scallops and shrimp, and heat until shrimp turns pink
and curls, about 5 minutes.

Per serving: 245 calories; 16 g protein; 2 g fat; 40 g carbohydrate

Pasta Primavera

Serves 4

(1 serving can substitute for 1 main-dish serving
in any dinner menu)

Sauce

2 teaspoons corn oil margarine
1 tablespoon flour
1 cup skim milk
½ cup defatted chicken broth

½ cup grated Parmesan cheese
1 teaspoon dried basil
¼ cup finely chopped parsley
½ teaspoon black pepper

Vegetable Mixture (see Unlimited Vegetable List
on page 90)

1 cup broccoli florets
1 cup snow peas, ends and
strings removed
1 cup zucchini, cut in round
slices

1 tablespoon finely chopped
white onion
1 large tomato, peeled, seeded,
and chopped
½ cup sliced mushrooms

8 ounces pasta (radiatore, vermicelli, macaroni, or shells),
cooked

To Make Sauce: Melt margarine in a 1-quart saucepan.
Add flour, blend well, and cook for 1 minute. Stir in milk
and stock, stirring constantly, and bring to a simmer, stirring,

until thickened. Add cheese, basil, parsley, and pepper and stir until cheese melts.

To Cook Vegetables: Steam broccoli, peas, and zucchini for 2 to 5 minutes in steamer rack, until tender-crisp. Sauté onion in a skillet coated with nonstick cooking spray. Add tomato and mushrooms to onion and cook for 4 minutes. Add steamed vegetables, tossing to combine.

To serve: Heap vegetables over pasta and pour sauce over vegetables.

Per serving: 336 calories; 16 g protein; 6 g fat; 57 g carbohydrate

Turkey Lasagne

Serves 8

(1 serving can substitute for 1 main-dish serving
in any dinner menu)

½ pound ground turkey
2 tablespoons finely chopped
  white onion
3 cups tomato sauce
1 teaspoon dried oregano
1 teaspoon dried basil
8 ounces lasagne noodles,
  cooked

2 cups low-fat cottage cheese,
  drained
1 cup shredded mozzarella
1 package chopped spinach,
  cooked and squeezed dry

Brown turkey and onion in a skillet coated with nonstick cooking spray. Add tomato sauce, oregano, and basil, and simmer for 20 minutes. Spread ⅓ cup of sauce in bottom of a baking pan. Layer ingredients starting with noodles, then cottage cheese, spinach, ½ cup mozzarella, and sauce. Repeat with a layer of noodles, cottage cheese, spinach, and sauce. Top with noodles and sauce. Bake the lasagne in a

350° oven for 25 minutes. Add the remaining mozzarella and bake 5 more minutes.

Per serving: 248 calories; 20 g protein; 8 g fat; 45 g carbohydrate

Shrimp and Vegetable Curry

Serves 6

(1 serving can substitute for 1 main-dish serving
in any dinner menu)

1 medium white onion, peeled and sliced thin
2 medium carrots, peeled and sliced thin
2 large white potatoes, peeled and cut in ¾-inch cubes
2 to 3 teaspoons curry powder
¼ teaspoon cinnamon

1 cup water
1½ cups fresh cauliflower pieces
2 cups canned tomatoes, broken
¼ cup raisins
½ pound shrimp, shelled and deveined

Sauté the onion in a large saucepan coated with nonstick cooking spray. Add the carrots, potatoes, curry powder, cinnamon, and water. Cover and simmer for 10 minutes. Add the cauliflower, tomatoes, and raisins, and bring to a simmer. Add shrimp; cover and simmer 5 more minutes. Serve over steamed white rice, using the quantity stated in the menu.

Per serving: 131 calories, 13 g protein; 1 g fat; 24 g carbohydrate

Crustless Vegetable with Rice Quiche

Serves 6

(1 serving can substitute for 1 bread in 1500- to 2500-calorie menus)

1 cup chopped white onion	2 cups cooked white rice
1 cup chopped mushrooms	2 eggs, beaten
2 cups chopped zucchini	⅔ cup low-fat cottage cheese
1 tomato, peeled, seeded, and chopped	¼ cup nonfat milk
¼ teaspoon dried basil	3 tablespoons Parmesan cheese
¼ teaspoon dried oregano	
1 teaspoon mild picante sauce (or Salsa from recipe on page 165)	

Coat a medium saucepan with nonstick cooking spray. Sauté onion, mushrooms, zucchini, and tomato until vegetables soften, about 5 minutes. Remove from heat and add the remaining ingredients, combining well. Pour into a 9-inch pie pan that has been spray-coated with nonstick cooking spray. Bake in a 350° oven for 25 to 30 minutes.

Per serving: 134 calories, 6 g protein; 3 g fat; 13 g carbohydrate

Vegetables

Generally, the Ultrafit Diets call for steamed fresh vegetables seasoned with herbs (see Mix and Match Herb Chart, page 161) or your favorite herb dressing or vinaigrette. To help you get started cooking steamed vegetables, I've created a table of vegetables, taken from the Unlimited Vegetable List on page 90, and given you the cooking times, whether you're cooking on a range or using a microwave. To cook in the microwave, add ⅛ cup water to cooking dish, unless I tell you differently.

To steam vegetables, use a steaming rack fitted inside a

pan that has a lid. Place vegetables on rack above 1 inch of water in the pan, and cover. Bring water to a boil. If you decide to use frozen vegetables, follow the directions on the package of the frozen food.

STEAMED VEGETABLE TABLE

FRESH VEGETABLE	AMOUNT	VEGETABLE PREPARATION	MICROWAVE TIME (MINUTES)	STEAMER TIME (MINUTES)
Artichokes	1	Wash thoroughly. Cut off top of each leaf.	7–8	20
	4		11–12	30
Asparagus	1 pound	Wash. Cut end stems off.	2–3	5
Beans: wax, green	1 pound	Wash, stem.	12–14	20
Beets	4 medium	Wash. Leave 1-inch stem on beets.	16–18	40–60
Broccoli	1 1½ pounds, whole	Wash. Remove leaves. Split.	9–10	8–10
Brussels Sprouts	1 pound	Wash. Remove wilted leaves.	8–9	10–20
Cabbage	½ medium head	Remove outer leaves.	5–6	20–30
Cauliflower	1 medium, cut in florets	Wash. Remove leaves, stem.	7–8	8–10
Celery	2½ cups 1-inch pieces	Clean stalks	8–9	5
Eggplant	1 medium, cut in cubes	Wash, peel.	5–6, 2 tbs. water	5
	1 medium, whole	Wash. Pierce with fork.	6–7, no water	5
Greens: beet, chard, collard, dandelion, spinach, turnip	1 pound	Wash. Stem.	6–7, no water	3–10

STEAMED VEGETABLE TABLE (cont.)

FRESH VEGETABLE	AMOUNT	VEGETABLE PREPARATION	MICROWAVE TIME (MINUTES)	STEAMER TIME (MINUTES)
Leeks	4	Wash. Leave 1-inch stem.	4–6	8–10
Mushrooms	½ pound, sliced	Wash.	2–4, 2 tbs. water	2–3
Okra	½ pound	Wash. Stem.	3–5	3–5
Onions	1 pound	Peel outer leaves.	6–7	10–15
Rutabagas	1 pound	Wash. Remove stems.	6–7, no water	10–15
Summer Squash: yellow, crookneck, patty pan, spaghetti, scalloped, zucchini	2 cups, sliced	Wash.	5–8, no water	3–5
Turnips	4 cups, cubed	Wash. Peel.	9–11	8–10

Substitute Vegetable and Grain Recipes

Sherried Mushroom and Broccoli Stir-Fry

Serves 8

(1 serving can substitute for 1 bread in the
1500- to 2500-calorie menus)

1 tablespoon corn oil margarine

¾ pound mushrooms, thinly sliced

1 pound fresh broccoli, trimmed and cut into bite-size pieces

1 pound carrots, peeled and julienned

½ cup thinly sliced scallions

1 tablespoon lemon juice

2 tablespoons dry sherry

1 teaspoon dried thyme

In a large skillet melt the margarine over medium heat. Add the vegetables and stir-fry until they are tender-crisp. Add the remaining ingredients, mix well and serve.

Per serving: 70 calories; 4 g protein; 1 g fat; 12 g carbohydrate

Baked Tomatoes

Serves 4

(1 serving can substitute for 1 bread in the
1500- to 2500-calorie menus)

4 medium tomatoes
½ teaspoon sugar
⅛ teaspoon dried oregano
⅛ teaspoon dried basil

½ cup crushed corn flakes
1 tablespoon corn oil
   margarine

Remove the stem ends of the tomatoes and scoop out some of the pulp. Chop the pulp and combine with the sugar, oregano, and basil. Return this mixture to the tomato shells. Combine the corn flakes with the margarine and sprinkle over the tomatoes. Bake in a 350° oven for 30 minutes.

Per serving: 86 calories; 2 g protein; 3 g fat; 13 g carbohydrate

Nutty Carrots

Serves 6

(1 serving can substitute for ½ bread in the
1500- to 2500-calorie menus)

⅓ cup water
1 tablespoon honey
2½ cups peeled, thinly sliced
  carrots
1½ teaspoons corn oil
  margarine

¼ teaspoon pepper
1 tablespoon finely ground
  pecans

Combine water, honey, carrots, margarine, and pepper in a
small saucepan. Cover and boil for 5 minutes. Remove the
cover and continue to boil until most of the liquid has evaporated, about 3 to 4 minutes. Drain and serve with ground
pecans sprinkled over the top.

Per serving: 48 calories; 1 g protein; 2 g fat; 8 g carbohydrate

Bulgur Pilaf

Serves 4

(1 serving can substitute for 1 bread in the
1500- to 2500-calorie menus)

¼ cup minced scallion
1 cup bulgur wheat
2 cups defatted chicken broth

½ teaspoon salt (omit if using
  salted broth)
¼ teaspoon thyme

Spray saucepan with nonstick cooking spray and sauté scallions until tender. Add remaining ingredients and bring to
a boil. Reduce heat to low, cover, and simmer for 15 minutes.

Per serving: 154 calories; 5 g protein; 1 g fat; 33 g carbohydrate

Herb Seasonings

Learn to mix herbs with other herbs, and match herbs with foods. If you haven't cooked with herbs before, experiment with them at first because they serve you and the foods you prepare in many ways. Herbs intensify, enhance, bring out the flavors of foods, even provide the most brilliant of flavors. When seasoning with herbs, using salt no longer becomes necessary. When using dried herbs, cut the amount to half that of fresh herbs.

Some herbs work together better than others. Certainly some herbs work better with certain foods. To get you started cooking with herbs, I've created a chart that matches herbs with herbs, and herbs with foods.

HERB	Compatible with:	
	Herb	*Food*
Basil	garlic, oregano, parsley, thyme	chicken, turkey, salads, tomatoes, broccoli, squash, eggplant, salad dressings
Chives	basil, garlic, parsley, tarragon	salads, cottage cheese, eggs, fish, chicken, breads, tomatoes
Cilantro	garlic, mint, parsley	salads, Mexican foods, Oriental foods, salsas, chicken, salad dressings
Dill	chives, fennel, mint, parsley	breads, fish, cucumbers, salads, salad dressings
Mint	coriander, garlic, parsley	vegetable salads, peas, desserts, fruit salads, rice

Oregano	basil, parsley, thyme	salads, cottage cheese, chicken, zucchini, cabbage, broccoli, salad dressings, tomatoes, eggplant
Parsley	basil, dill, garlic, oregano, thyme	salads, cottage cheese, chicken, potatoes, eggs, zucchini, soups, tomatoes, salad dressings, seafood
Rosemary	garlic, parsley, sage, thyme	chicken, salad dressings, fruit salads, tomatoes, cauliflower, green beans
Sage	parsley, rosemary, thyme	stuffing for poultry, egg soufflés, tomatoes, cottage cheese
Tarragon	chives, oregano, parsley, rosemary, thyme	chicken, salads, salad dressings, soups, eggs, mushrooms, sauerkraut
Thyme	basil, dill, garlic, oregano, parsley, rosemary, sage	fish, chicken, salads, salad dressings, broccoli, summer squashes, seafoods, soups, eggplant, beets, onions

Salads: Toss Your Own

Create your own salad from any of these vegetables taken from the Unlimited Vegetable List on page 90. Dice, slice, chop, tear as you prefer. Remember to use fresh or dried herbs to season your salads. (See the Mix-and-Match Herb Chart on page 161.)

Artichoke Hearts
Bamboo Shoots
Bean Sprouts
Beans: green and yellow
Beets
Broccoli Florets
Cabbage
Cauliflower Florets
Celery
Chicory
Chinese Cabbage
Cucumber

Endive
Fennel
Mushrooms
Onions
Peppers: green, yellow, red bell, chili, banana
Radishes
Romaine
Scallions
Spinach
Summer Squashes
Tomatoes

Dressings and Relishes

Herb Dressing

Makes ¼ cup (4 tablespoons)

1 garlic clove
1 tablespoon, chopped parsley
¼ cup favorite herb vinegar (lemon, tarragon, basil)

Juice of ½ lemon
½ teaspoon of your favorite herb (tarragon, basil, thyme)

Blend in blender or food processor. Use 1 tablespoon over salad or vegetables.

Nutrient content is negligible.

Cilantro Dressing

Makes ¾ cup (12 tablespoons)

1 cup lightly packed fresh cilantro leaves
1 cup lightly packed fresh mint
   leaves

2 green chili peppers, stemmed
   and seeded
1 garlic clove
¼ cup lemon vinegar

Place ingredients in blender and puree. Use at once or place
in sealed jar and refrigerate. Use 1 tablespoon over salads,
sliced tomatoes, vegetables, or over sautéed or poached fish.

Nutrient content is negligible.

Vinaigrette Dressing

Makes ⅛ cup (2 tablespoons)

1 teaspoon Dijon-style mustard
1 tablespoon finely chopped
   shallots
1 garlic clove, minced

1 tablespoon finely minced
   parsley
1 tablespoon red wine vinegar
Freshly ground pepper to taste

Place ingredients in a jar and shake. Use immediately or
seal and refrigerate. Use 1 tablespoon over salads or
vegetables.

Nutrient content is negligible.

Salsa

Makes 1½ cups (24 tablespoons)

1 medium fresh tomato
1 medium white onion
3 fresh green chilis, hot or
   regular
1 tablespoon finely chopped cilantro or parsley

½ medium carrot, peeled and
   chopped
1 tablespoon red wine vinegar
2 to 4 tablespoons water
Twist of freshly ground pepper

Mince all ingredients very fine, either with a sharp knife or in a blender or food processor. Do not chop so finely that you turn the ingredients into mush. The salsa tastes best when served fresh, up to three hours. Beyond that, cover and refrigerate. Use 1 tablespoon over salads, vegetables, chicken, or fish for flavor addition.

Nutrient content is negligible.

Corn Relish

Makes 2 cups (¼ cup per serving)

1 cup frozen corn, cooked according to package
   directions
1 medium firm tomato, diced
¼ cup diced dill pickle
½ green bell pepper, diced

2 tablespoons apple cider
   vinegar
1 teaspoon mustard seed
½ teaspoon freshly ground
   pepper
¼ teaspoon celery seed

Mix ingredients. Use at once, or cover and chill in refrigerator.

Per serving: 21 calories; 1 g protein; 0 g fat; 5 g carbohydrate

Dill-Mustard Sauce for Fish

Makes ¾ cup (12 tablespoons)

¼ cup apple cider vinegar
2 tablespoons Dijon-style
  mustard
2 teaspoons dried dill

1½ teaspoons dry mustard
1½ teaspoons sugar
¼ cup water

Shake ingredients in closed pint jar. Refrigerate. Use 1 tablespoon over fish.

Nutrient content is negligible.

Desserts

Fruit Salad

Serves 4

1 Red Delicious apple, cored
  and diced
10 white seedless grapes, cut in
  half
½ cup fresh strawberries,
  stemmed and cut in half

½ small cantaloupe, peeled,
  seeded, and cubed
1 medium orange, peeled and
  diced
Juice of ½ lemon

Mix fruit in a bowl, sprinkle with lemon juice, and toss. Chill for 1 hour.

Per serving: 85 calories; 1 g protein; 0 g fat; 22 g carbohydrate

Banana "Ice Cream"

Serves 4

2 large ripe bananas, peeled,   6 to 7 tablespoons skim milk
   sliced, and frozen

Process the banana slices in the food processor or blender until grainy, about 1 minute. Add the milk, a few tablespoons at a time, and process until smooth and creamy. Serve at once.

Per serving: 58 calories; 1 g protein; 0 g fat; 14 g carbohydrate

Jelly Roll

Serves 12

3 eggs   1 teaspoon baking powder
1 cup sugar   ¼ teaspoon salt
5 tablespoons water   Confectioners' sugar, divided
1 teaspoon vanilla   1 cup blackberry jam
¾ cup all-purpose flour

Beat the eggs until they thicken, about 5 minutes. Gradually add the sugar while continuing to beat mixture. With mixer on low speed, slowly add the water and vanilla. Gradually add the combined flour, baking powder, and salt. Beat until smooth.

Pour the batter into a wax paper-lined 10 × 15-inch jelly roll pan and bake in a 375° oven for 12 minutes. Sprinkle a clean cloth towel with sifted confectioners' sugar and invert the hot cake onto it. Remove the wax paper and, starting with the narrow end, roll cake and towel together; cool on rack, about 45 minutes. Unroll and spread with blackberry jam. Roll up. Sprinkle lightly with confectioners' sugar and slice.

Per serving: 177 calories; 3 g protein; 1 g fat; 47 g carbohydrate

Fluffy Lime Pudding

Serves 6

1 tablespoon unflavored gelatin
  softened in 1 tablespoon cold
  water
½ cup sugar
¼ cup fresh lime juice

1 teaspoon grated lime rind
1 cup boiling water
½ cup cold water
½ cup whole powdered milk
½ cup iced water

In a mixing bowl, combine the softened gelatin, sugar, lime juice, and rind with boiling water. Stir until the sugar is dissolved. Add the cold water and chill in the refrigerator until very firm. In another bowl, mix the powdered milk with iced water. Beat at high speed until fluffy. Combine whipped milk with gelatin mixture and beat in mixer until fluffy. Chill until firm.

Per serving: 106 calories; 4 g protein; 0 g fat; 18 g carbohydrate

Peach Crisp

Serves 8

4 cups sliced peaches: fresh,
  peeled, canned, or frozen
1 cup raisins
⅓ cup honey
1 teaspoon lemon juice

1 tablespoon cinnamon
¾ cup oatmeal
¼ cup whole wheat flour
2 tablespoons melted corn oil
  margarine

Combine the peaches, raisins, honey, lemon juice, and cinnamon in a bowl and set aside for 30 minutes so flavors can blend. Spread the mixture in a 8 × 8-inch baking dish coated with nonstick cooking spray. Combine the oatmeal, flour, and margarine and sprinkle over the peach mixture. Bake in a 325° oven for 30 to 40 minutes.

Per serving: 175 calories; 2 g protein; 3 g fat; 37 g carbohydrate

Cinnamon-Baked Apples

Serves 4

4 medium tart apples (Rome, MacIntosh), cored
4 teaspoons brown sugar

2 tablespoons Butter Buds
1 teaspoon cinnamon

Place the apples in a baking dish. Mix the brown sugar, Butter Buds, and cinnamon. Fill each cavity with brown sugar mixture. Bake for 1 hour in a 350° oven, or microwave for 10 minutes on high power.

Per serving: 114 calories; 0 g protein; 1 g fat; 29 g carbohydrate

> Man takes a vacation from exercise between
> the ages of 25 and 30 and pays for it
> the rest of his life.
> —PAUL DUDLEY WHITE, M.D.

CHAPTER NINE

The Value of Exercise

Personally, I love to exercise. At the end of the day when I leave the office, I go directly to my gym where I work out. After an hour, a sense of peace fills me. Frankly, I consider exercise the best tranquilizer on the market. It doesn't have to cost a cent either. At first, it may cost you a few stiff muscles, or a sore fanny. You are worth that!

Exercise can prolong your life. Medical study after medical study shows this. I consider exercise so important that I insist all my patients exercise regularly. That doesn't mean you have to dress yourself in iridescent leotards and dance to Little Richard's pounding music.

I think I know how you might feel when I issue the statement that to reach the Ultrafit State you must exercise. I've seen the same look on my patients' faces when I go into my exercise lecture. They roll their eyes back, heave a sigh, and give me that indulgent look. Yet, in the Ultrafit State, you experience the fullness of your life.

Remember Edna? Perhaps you remember her from Chapter One. At age 62, Edna suffered from severe degenerative arthritis of the knees. She weighed 265 pounds, stood five feet, four inches, and walked with a cane.

Edna had never exercised in her entire life. She didn't for many reasons, one of which involved her poor self-image that she'd developed over the years as she gradually gained weight.

When I placed Edna on the Ultrafit Amino Acid Diet, I told her we needed to work out an exercise program tailored to her. She looked at me in disbelief. "Doctor, I've never exercised in my entire life. With the arthritis in my knees, how do you expect me to do anything? I can't walk without my cane."

I told Edna that exercise would help so many of her problems that we could not afford to leave it out of her program. I told her that medical research showed that persons with degenerative arthritis who did not exercise actually got worse. Their disease increased.

Walking, through the hydraulic effect on the joints, forces nutrients into the damaged cartilage. This helps the healing process. "But it hurts when I walk, Doctor," Edna said.

I pointed out to Edna that, yes, at first when she started walking, she did hurt. As she walked, and got warmed up, the pain would become less and less. If she didn't exercise, she'd experience even worse pain in the future.

She and I designed a treadmill exercise program for her that she could do in her home. On the treadmill, part of her weight was supported on her arms and shoulders. That relieved some of the stress to her knee joints caused by her great weight.

An amazing thing happened. As Edna's weight dropped rapidly, and her percent body fat dropped rapidly, she developed muscle tissue. The muscle tissue helped support her frame, much like a scaffolding supports a weak building. The pain in her knees became less and less.

Ten weeks passed. Edna lost 48 pounds. At this point, she walked into my office without her cane, a broad smile on her face. "When can I start walking with my husband in the neighborhood?" she asked.

In our next step, we tailored her exercise program to allow her to walk in her home for 20 minutes each day. At this point, it took all her energy to walk those 20 minutes.

One year later, Edna walked each day with her husband in the neighborhood for 30 minutes. Currently, she weighs 165 pounds and rarely needs to take an aspirin for her arthritis.

Does this sound dramatic? It's commonplace for those who get motivated and exercise.

Edna had so many problems that exercise helped. I'd like for you to take a closer look at her situation.

Initially, Edna had elevated blood pressure and took a number of medications for that condition. She had an elevated cholesterol level, too.

Exercise, in addition to the diet, lowered her blood pressure and cholesterol levels. Medical science still doesn't know how this phenomenon operates. We just know it happens.

Medical science does know the effect exercise has on Edna's metabolism. Beginning in your middle to late 20s, your metabolic rate begins to show a steady decline. People who exercise do not show this decline. Each decade your metabolic rate declines further. Again, people who exercise do not show this decline.

At age 62, Edna's metabolic rate had dropped so low that when she ate 1000 calories a day, she gained weight.

By now you should be well-acquainted with another reason Edna gained weight no matter what she ate. She had almost no muscle tissue, and almost no mitochondria. With her fuel-burning units gone, she could not hope to lose weight if she did not exercise.

Edna suffered from diabetes and took oral agents to control her blood sugar. The exercise increased the muscle tissue and thus increased the number of insulin receptors her body made. Exercise also increased the sensitivity of the individual receptors to the effects of insulin.

The result of her exercise? Edna no longer suffers from diabetes. I doubt if she ever will again.

Edna did not like to admit she had suffered depression most of her life. I pointed out to her that it influenced her eating, her self-image, her lack of confidence in her ability to lose weight. I told her we needed to talk about it.

Much to her surprise, she discovered that she always felt better after she exercised. I explained to her that when she exercised, her body released certain hormones, called endorphins, that trigger a feeling of euphoria when infused into the brain tissue from the bloodstream.

In psychiatric hospitals, you now see exercise programs used as part of a patient's therapy. Exercise proves more effective than medication in the treatment of depression.

Aerobic Versus Anaerobic Exercise

We have Dr. Kenneth Cooper to thank for making the words "aerobic" and "anaerobic" household words. He became our Pied Piper of exercise and his books continue to serve as sources of inspiration. He got the people of this country out of their homes and into exercise programs in numbers never before seen.

It's important to understand what these two forms of exercise do.

Aerobic exercise burns fat and builds mitochondria.

Anaerobic exercise builds mitochondria, but does not burn fat.

To reach the Ultrafit State, I recommend that you engage in aerobic exercise. Let me explain the differences between these two forms of exercise.

Aerobic means, literally, in the presence of oxygen. When you perform aerobic exercise, you burn fuel in the presence of oxygen. Your body will burn some glycogen stores in your muscle, but primarily you use fat stores as a source of energy.

Why?

Fat burns in the presence of oxygen.

Aerobic exercise places demands on your body that cannot be met by the glycogen stores in your muscle and in your liver. This causes you to use stored fat as an energy source for the exercise.

This effect begins fifteen to twenty minutes after starting an aerobic exercise. The longer you exercise, the more your body shifts to using stored fat as an energy source.

Aerobic exercise offers another bonus. Long after you've stopped exercising, your body continues to burn stored fat for several hours. That is, it continues to burn stored fat if you do not eat excessive calories, particularly in the form of fat.

Aerobic exercise speeds your metabolic rate, both immediately and through the production of mitochondria.

If you build an exercise program for yourself over a period of time, and stay with that program on a regular basis, your body adapts itself to using stored fat more easily. The longer you stay with your regular exercise program, the more efficient your body becomes in burning fat.

Anaerobic exercise does not require the presence of oxygen to be performed. This kind of exercise does not use fat stores to any great extent. Anaerobic exercise, which includes short bursts of exercise, uses glycogen or sugar stores in the muscles and liver for energy. The burning of glycogen can take place without the presence of oxygen, hence the term "anaerobic." Because anaerobic activity lasts a short period of time, the body does not mobilize fat to provide energy for the activity.

What's Aerobic?

Aerobic exercises include walking, jogging, aerobic dancing, vigorous calisthenics, rope jumping, cross-country skiing, swimming, stair climbing, rowing, and bicycling.

I'm sure you know of other aerobic forms of exercise. Almost any type of movement can be turned into an aerobic exercise as long as you perform it repetitively and rhythmically, and it causes you to breathe harder.

What may be aerobic for you will not be for another person. Edna, when she first started on her program, found that raising her arms over her head while sitting in a chair caused her to become breathless and accelerated her heart rate. This simple exercise was an aerobic activity for Edna but, depending on your condition, it may not be for you.

What's Anaerobic?

Anaerobic exercises include touch football, weight lifting, sprinting, downhill skiing, bowling, handball, and tennis.

Anaerobic exercise involves activity that causes you to make any sudden, jerky, nonrepetitive body motions. These motions burn glycogen in the muscle tissue and the liver. If you participate in these activities long enough, and do not eat, you will eventually start burning your fat stores. However, you must engage in these activities several hours before you start burning fat.

Calorie-Burning Rates

Occasionally, I hear one of my patients tell me, "Doc, the exercise won't do me any good because I'm a slow metabolizer. There's no way I can exercise that much to catch up with the normal person."

When I talk about someone being a slow or fast metabolizer, I'm talking about their *basal* metabolism. Basal metabolism measures how fast a person burns calories in the basal state. The basal state means the calorie-burning rate at total rest. Total rest means the person lies quietly in bed, but is not asleep.

Exercise affects a person at the same rate, whether that person has a slow or fast basal metabolism. This means that if you have a slow basal metabolic rate, exercise increases your metabolic rate. If you have a fast metabolic rate, exercise increases your metabolic rate.

What things influence the basal metabolic rate, in addition to your genetics? Exercise has the most dramatic effect. Short bursts of exercise can accelerate the basal metabolic rate to as much as 10,000 percent for a few seconds.

Let's look at the basal metabolic rate, that is, the rate taken when you are at complete rest and awake, for various kinds of people.

The average woman, who weighs 120 pounds, metabolizes approximately 50 calories per hour at her basal rate. This rate changes with various levels of activity. For example, if she goes to sleep, she uses only 35 calories an hour. If she sits in a chair, her metabolism rate speeds up to 75 calories an hour.

The average man, who weighs 150 pounds, metabolizes approximately 77 calories per hour at his basal rate. This rate changes with various levels of activity. For example, if he goes to sleep, he uses 65 calories an hour. If he sits in a chair, his metabolic rate speeds up to 100 calories an hour.

Why are these numbers important to you? Simple math, my friends. Figure out the number of calories you burn in a completely passive state. I've made this easy for you. Look on page 56 where I've given you the number of calories that the average and slow metabolizing woman and man use per pound of body weight. This figure represents the usual number of calories that the average sedentary person uses.

Then figure out the number of calories you consume during the day. Now subtract the two numbers. Notice how many calories you need to burn to make the numbers equal?

Next, look at the number of calories burned in the different kinds of exercise. On page 178 I've listed the number of calories burned by engaging in different kinds of exercise so that you can choose how you want to burn your excess calories.

A well-trained athelete can increase the metabolic rate 2000 percent for several minutes. For the nonathlete, the figure is still impressive at 1000 percent above basal with vigorous exercise, and a respectable rise with an exercise such as a brisk walking.

Let me get you started calculating your calorie use, so that you can compare the calories you use at your basal metabolic rate and at your sedentary rate. This will help you understand the difference between your basal rate and your metabolic rate with activities added.

If the average nonobese woman, who weighs 120 pounds, lies in bed for 24 hours, sleeping 8 hours and lying quietly at rest for the other 16 hours, she will use about 1080 calories. This represents her basal rate. If that woman eats three reasonable meals during those 24 hours, digesting the food will add 150 calories. If she sits in a chair 16 of those hours and sleeps 8 and does nothing but eat three meals, she will burn approximately 1630 calories in 24 hours.

If the average nonobese man, who weighs 150 pounds, lies in bed 24 hours, sleeping 8 hours and lying quietly at rest for the other 16 hours, he will use about 1700 calories. This represents his basal rate. If that man eats three reasonable meals during those 24 hours, digesting the food will add 200 calories. If he sits in a chair for 16 hours and sleeps 8 hours and does nothing but eat three meals, he will burn approximately 2300 calories.

For the slow metabolizer, cut the figures for the average person by as much as one half. Sitting and eating three meals a day, for the slow metabolizing woman or man, uses 800 to 1000 calories per day.

What can you expect if you exercise? This table gives approximate figures for the amount of calories burned by any person, no matter what their basal metabolic rate. Now that I've said that, there is one exception. The first two activities listed, sleeping and sitting at rest, only apply to the average metabolizer.

ACTIVITY	CALORIES PER HOUR	
	Woman	*Man*
Sleeping	35	65
Sitting at rest	75	100
Standing relaxed	80	105
Dressing and undressing	88	118
Typing	105	140
Walking slowly (2.5 mph)	150	200
Carpentry	180	240
Active exercise—tennis, light calisthenics	220	290
Intense exercise—aerobic dancing, vigorous calisthenics, jumping rope	340	450
Sawing wood	360	480
Swimming	375	500
Jogging (5.3 mph)	430	570
Walking rapidly (5.3 mph)	490	650
Walking up stairs	825	1100

Remember, the effects of exercise last long after you complete the exercise. You can measure your increased metabolic rate several hours after you've completed your exercise.

Exercise that uses your larger muscles burns greater amounts of fat. For example, exercise that uses the legs and back burns calories at a much greater rate, thanks to your increased number of mitochondria in these larger muscles. That's why I try, at all times, to get my patients on walking programs.

Other Metabolic Influences

Other factors increase your metabolic rate. I've designed the Ultrafit Diet plans to take advantage of them.

Eating food actually accelerates your metabolic rate. After a meal, your metabolic rate increases. To a slight degree, this happens during the chemical reactions associated with the digestion and absorption of food. Mainly, it results from direct stimulation of the cellular metabolic reactions by certain of the amino acids derived from the proteins in foods you just ate. We call this the specific dynamic action of protein, or the thermogenic effect of protein.

Remember, foods other than protein—melons and berries—have this effect on your metabolism. Let's suppose you have an average weight and basal rate. If you started eating your 1500 calories in the form of strawberries, you'd start losing weight. It takes more calories to digest, absorb, and process the strawberries than your body actually derives from the berries.

Metabolic rate declines with age. Children, relative to size, use twice as many calories as their parents.

Thyroid hormone accelerates the metabolic rate. But let me make an important point here. Thyroid hormone has a number of other physiologic effects on the body as well. Thyroid consumption can *endanger* your health if you try to cheat Mother Nature and your genes by taking more of the hormone than your body needs.

Anxiety increases your metabolic rate. This probably happens through the increased supply of adrenaline, a hormone known to increase the mobilization of fat stores and calorie burning in your body. You probably know someone who endures high anxiety. This person wrings their hands constantly and never stops moving.

The male sex hormone, testosterone, and, to a lesser degree, the female hormone, estrogen, stimulate your calorie-burning rate. This, besides the differences in genetic makeup, probably explains why women, in general, burn calories at a slower rate than men.

The temperature of your surroundings greatly affects your metabolic rate. If you live in a colder climate, you burn calories at a faster rate than if you live in a warmer climate. If you exercise in cold weather, you get a double benefit. Cross-country skiiers burn calories at one of the highest rates.

Tailoring Your Exercise

I often see the "yes, but" syndrome emerge when I talk to patients about exercise. Yes, but Doctor, I can't exercise because I hurt . . . live in an unsafe area . . . it's too hot . . . it's too cold . . . it's too rainy . . . it's too dark when I get home . . . I'm too tired . . . I don't have time . . . I'm embarrassed . . . I'm afraid of dogs . . . and, finally, "I hate to exercise."

I find that until a person experiences the benefits of exercise, he or she cannot know the wonders of exercise. I know that if I can get a patient to exercise regularly for three months, that person gets hooked on exercise. The patient feels so much better that the positive effect reinforces the experience.

For those who resist exercise, I ask, "What do you enjoy most? Choose that exercise. Exercise must become a daily part of your life, just like getting dressed, eating, brushing your teeth. If you believe you can live a healthy life without exercise, you're wrong."

What exercise do I recommend most?

I consider rapid walking the most perfect form of aerobic exercise. It accelerates your metabolic rate, increases your muscle tissue, and prevents damage to your joints.

I also suggest, if you can swing it financially, that you buy a piece of exercise equipment that suits your needs. When you can't walk outside, up stairwells at work, or jog, you can exercise indoors in the privacy of your home.

If you believe that you live in an area that does not allow you to walk outside, consider buying a treadmill. If that doesn't interest you, think about investing in a cross-country skiing machine that forces you to use your arms and legs simultaneously. If you won't consider either of these, think of buying a bicycle exerciser or a rowing machine.

Each of us invests in equipment or items we consider necessary to our happiness and health. You may buy a television set, a stereo system, a piece of furniture, or a coat that you believe enhances your life. I'm telling you that your investment in exercise equipment fits that category. Exercise *prolongs* and *enhances* your life. I believe that's worth $200 to $500.

Sometimes I suggest that a particular patient develop a buddy system with a friend. This particular kind of patient has a hard time motivating himself or herself. They have up and down days. On the down days, they simply cannot get their mind wrapped around exercise.

The buddy system really helps. Bodybuilders use it with a training partner. When you don't feel like training, the buddy gets you going and motivated.

If you don't have a buddy you feel you can ask to join you in exercising, consider joining a fitness center. We're all social animals, some more than others. At a fitness center you can find people whose enthusiasm infects you.

Many recreation centers in larger cities have excellent dancing programs. I have several patients who go square dancing and ballroom dancing twice a week. Dancing offers an excellent aerobic exercise.

If you live in a large city and commute to work by bus or train, park your car two miles from where you board the bus or train, and briskly walk the distance. I know several people who walk these distances morning and evening during the work week. The exercise snaps them awake in the morning and calms them in the evening.

Frequently Asked Questions

What is the best time of day to exercise?

If you have your choice, exercise early in the morning. If you exercise early in the morning, you've already completed one of your most important tasks. You stand less chance of having your schedule interrupted or using your schedule as an excuse not to exercise. You take advantage of your metabolism by getting your metabolic rate running at a faster rate.

Athletes who become involved in peak performances find that they reach their optimal physical capacity at approximately 4 P.M. However, because most aerobic exercises do not involve peak performances, I suggest you exercise in the morning.

How soon after eating a meal can I exercise?

If you plan to exercise vigorously, that is, anaerobically, wait one and a half to two hours. If you plan to walk rapidly or engage in any of the other aerobic exercises, wait 30 minutes to an hour. If you have underlying heart disease, wait two hours.

How soon can I eat after exercising?

Wait 20 to 30 minutes after completing your exercise to eat a meal.

Once I start exercising, must I continue for the rest of my life?

Yes. But not for the reason you may think. Perhaps you've heard the old wives' tale that if you stop exercising your muscles will turn to flab. That won't happen. You will lose muscle tissue. Over time, your loss of mitochondria cuts your calorie-burning capacity. If you continue to eat calories at the rate you did when you exercised, you will add fat.

Do women risk building large muscles if they lift weights?

In general, no. Building large muscles has more to do with your hormone level than your rate of exercise. Some women produce large amounts of testosterone. These women can, indeed, build big muscles. Women who produce normal amounts of testosterone and estrogen need not worry about building bulging muscles. Their hormones prevent this from happening.

To sum up, everyone needs muscle tissue. Everyone needs to exercise.

Exercise and Sleep

Exercise provides the best sleeping potion known to man. Medical studies show that moderate exercise increases the most restful phases of sleep at night. Too much or too little exercise can cause insomnia.

Vigorous exercise, for as short a period of time as 15 minutes, can help you control your hunger.

> Guilt is a useless emotion. What we all need is a
> healthy sense of conscience.
> —MARLON BRANDO

CHAPTER TEN

The Pig-Out Meal

While attending medical school, I watched Sesame Street
with my son. He and I would identify with the various characters. I loved Grover, the hip character whose abundance
of blue hair I envied. But I identified with the Cookie
Monster.

I am a cookie monster.

I can say, "No thank you," to cakes, pies, and ice cream.
I cannot resist cookies. The cheapest store-bought brands of
cookies satisfy me. My wife, loving spouse that she is, always
kept me supplied with fresh-baked cookies after we married.

One day, while in medical residency, I awoke to the fact
that I am addicted to sweets. I had to find a solution to my
problem.

I discovered a secret weapon to control my cookie monster
trait. If I controlled my eating impulses for a full week, I
allowed myself one meal in which I could eat everything I
wanted, and in quantities that filled my greatest fantasies.

I called this the "pig-out meal."

I stopped eating sweets cold turkey. This system worked
so well for me that I now recommend it to my patients. I've
made it a part of the Ultrafit Maintenance Diet.

Here's how and why it works.

If you eat large amounts of unrefined sugar at a single
sitting, you will not absorb all that sugar. Part of the sugar
remains undigested in your gastrointestinal tract. In fact, you

may experience diarrhea if you haven't eaten unrefined sugar during the week.

Your body stores much of the sugar in your liver as glycogen. Again, if you do not call upon your glycogen reserves, your body will excrete the excess if you do not repeat the process more often than once a week.

In other words, your body adapts to what it does regularly. If you constantly bombard your body with excess sugar, your body will find a way to use it; most probably it will store the sugar as fat. If you take sugar infrequently, your body senses the exception and refuses to change its metabolic process for something that happens so infrequently.

You may experience a weight gain of two or three pounds the day after your pig-out. Don't worry. You did not gain body fat.

Here's why.

For each molecule of glucose that your body takes in, it takes in two molecules of water. The weight gain after your pig-out meal comes mostly from water. Over the next 24 to 36 hours, you will discover that your weight falls back to its previous level. You will eliminate the water through urination.

For the past ten years, I've been faithful to the pig-out principles. I have been known to eat up to two dozen chocolate chip cookies at one sitting. I actually ate a whole buttermilk pie on one occasion. The list of my indulgences on pig-out night is disgustingly long.

You will want to work out a similar program if you feel you need to indulge in excessive eating on occasion. Here are the ground rules.

Pig-Out Principles

1. The pig-out meal applies only if you follow the Ultrafit Maintenance Diet. You cannot eat the pig-out meal when you follow the Ultrafit Amino Acid Diet and

Ultrafit Reducing Diet. When you follow a reduced-calorie diet, if you suddenly load your system with excess sugar, the sudden shock to your system causes too much stress. Too, you can benefit by staying on a reduced-calorie diet by training yourself to eat smaller servings and certain foods.

2. You can eat only one pig-out meal per week.

3. You must select the same mealtime and the same day each week for your pig-out meal.

However, if a holiday, birthday, or special occasion occurs during the week, you may substitute the special-event meal for your pig-out meal. You may substitute no other meals. For example, if you find yourself at a banquet or at a friend's house, you must not eat the sugar-loaded dessert unless it is your pig-out mealtime.

If your aunt brings you a freshly baked pecan pie on Monday, and your pig-out meal falls on Saturday, you must freeze the pie and save it until Saturday, or give it away.

4. If you miss your pig-out meal, congratulations. Your self-discipline works. Don't weaken and fantasize that you can double up on your pig-out meals the next week to make up for your missed pig-out event. Stay focused on your goal to become healthy.

5. Try to confine your pig-out foods to those loaded with sugar. Work to not eat foods loaded with fat. You can bring on a heart attack when you load your body with fatty foods. Every Christmas or Thanksgiving, if I'm in town, I can always plan on being called to the hospital to attend at least one patient, sometimes more, suffering a heart attack from having eaten excessive fat at the holiday meal.

Here's why.

The fat globules found in your bloodstream after eating large amounts of fatty foods can literally block some of the small vessels in your circulatory system and precipitate a heart attack.

You stand a greater risk of this happening if you have a known history of coronary artery disease.

6. Do not feel guilty about eating your pig-out meal. Guilt does not belong at the table with you and your pig-out meal. You worked for your pig-out meal, you earned it. Now look forward to it, and enjoy it.

Each of us harbors a Joan of Arc deep within us. Even if she's a tiny Joan of Arc, she still represents the martyr in us. The pig-out meal helps to relieve your martyr needs, even small ones. The meal serves, too, to help you get better acquainted with why you eat, and how you feel about eating.

Eating Games

I see patients who play games with the way they eat to excess. Too frequently, I find that this kind of person eats to excess as a form of self-punishment. The patient plays the game without being aware.

Their pleasure does not come from the food itself. I recognize that the patient finds pleasure in telling me what a bad person he or she is. These people brag about their lack of self-control.

Wanda had this problem. Wanda first came to me when she weighed 208 pounds. She stood five feet, two inches tall. Five years later, she weighed 198.

Wanda suffers from high blood pressure and angina pectoris, pain in the chest due to blockage in her coronary arteries.

Wanda exercises discipline. She always makes her medical appointments. When I suggest a date, she volunteers to come at an earlier date.

She comes in and says, as she smiles, "Boy, am I going to get chewed out today." Then she gives me a list of all her eating indiscretions during the week: ice cream, candy, Hostess Twinkies, Cokes.

I recognized from the beginning that Wanda wanted me to punish her for being a bad person. She wanted to hand me control over her life. We talked about this. I asked her, "Why don't you like yourself? Giving me control over your diet won't work. Your coming in here and bragging about your lack of self-discipline has not changed your eating habits."

She admitted she did not understand what caused her to walk into my office and announce, "You're going to be so mad at me. I'm such a pig." Wanda needed psychological counseling. I could not control her excessive eating. She began to work through her problems with a clinical psychologist. We feel hopeful for her progress.

If you play eating games, you need to become aware of them before you can take action. We all play games. The pig-out meal offers an eating game that you consciously control.

Pigs and Discipline

You may think that a contradiction exists in a diet plan that allows a pig-out meal while insisting on self-control. I believe they work together.

Let me explain.

The pig-out meal represents a reward system. It offers a ritualized event that you can look forward to week after week. It puts you in control of your own decision-making process when you exercise self-discipline for one week.

I do not believe that you or I can or should eliminate sweets from our diets. Sweets do have a place in your meals. On the Ultrafit Maintenance Diet the pig-out meal becomes that place for them. It brings you pleasure while you safeguard your health.

You safeguard your health when you eliminate the chronic sugar loads that bring on disease. Medical studies show that chronic excesses of simple sugars lead to medical conditions such as diabetes and elevated blood lipids, cholesterol, and triglycerides.

Let me make the distinction, again, between simple and complex carbohydrates. Simple carbohydrates come in the form of table sugar and honey. You want to eliminate these from your day-to-day eating, except for your pig-out meal.

Complex carbohydrates belong in your Ultrafit Diet. Breads, vegetables, grain cereals, fruits, and pasta represent complex carbohydrates. Ultimately, your body converts these foods to glucose to be burned by your mitochondria.

The pig-out meal allows you to regain control over your life and your eating patterns. Too many times, stress in our day-to-day existence leads to a sense of loss of control. The pig-out meal, and the self-discipline needed to stick to the day-to-day eating that allows a special meal, can put order back into your life.

It's not the single meal of sweets that causes you to gain weight. It's the day-after-day consumption of sweets that puts on pounds.

The average candy bar contains 240 calories. Eating a single candy bar a day for one year will produce 25 pounds of body fat.

We are never so happy nor so unhappy
as we imagine.
—LA ROCHEFOUCAULD

CHAPTER ELEVEN

Stress and Coping: Unleashing Your Attitude

Your attitude can change your life. You've probably read about the most dramatic changes. Medical study after study has documented people who actually changed the course of diseases that ravaged their bodies. Patients have overcome cancer through a positive mental attitude.

These people changed a negative situation with a positive attitude.

I want you to start with a positive attitude. You must incorporate a positive attitude into your life on your way to the Ultrafit State. I'm going to show you different ways you can manage your life with a positive attitude.

Unfortunately, medical scientists shy away from this aspect of health simply because you can't put a number on it. We can put numbers on blood counts, cholesterol, blood pressure, cell activity, weight gains and losses. But we can't put a number on your enthusiasm.

Enthusiasm belongs in your life. Without enthusiasm, you cannot achieve the Ultrafit State or a life-time weight control discipline.

I asked you to go to your doctor and get your blood cholesterol, blood pressure, and percent body fat measured. Only you can measure your attitude and your level of enthusiasm.

Cycle of Moods

Every spring, I see hordes of people go on diets. This country abounds in enthusiastic devotees of the newest diet plan. Why? What can you learn from this recurring event?

I believe that we as individuals, and collectively as a society, go through cycles of enthusiasm. All of life moves through cycles, and the seasons represent one example. Your moods cycle just as do the seasons.

You don't need to be a psychologist to know that you experience swings in mood. I prefer to call them circles of moods because, if you examine your moods carefully, you can find them revolving, from happiness to sadness, from excitement to lethargy, with degress of variation between.

I have them. You have them. My patients have them. You must accept and understand the inevitability of these cyclical mood changes in your quest for long-term weight control and the Ultrafit State.

Why do I want you to spend most of your time in the upbeat cycle of your mood? It's simple. Enthusiastic individuals burn calories at a faster rate than depressed or despondent ones, primarily because your metabolic rate speeds up when you experience joy and happiness. Here's how you can control and change the speed of your cyclical moods.

Exercise

When you wake up, start the day by asking yourself where you stand in the cycle of moods. If you don't know, exercise to get yourself thinking. What kind of exercise? You picked the kind that best fits you; do it now.

Let me repeat how exercise alters mood. Research has shown that exercise produces a family of hormones called endorphins. These small compounds elevate your mood. No one knows just how they achieve this. We know it happens. Use exercise during the day or in the evening to elevate your mood. Make your body work for you by unleashing its chemistry.

Music

I know of no one who can listen to Beethoven's Ninth Symphony and not get excited. Music remains key to the human spirit. Music speaks to the family of man. Every culture has its music.

Rulers used music to inspire soldiers going into battle. Doctors use music in psychiatric hospitals to treat depression. The recording industry has created an entirely new line of recordings in mood and New Wave music to alter your mood.

When I feel my enthusiasm falling, I turn on Mozart, Bach, Beethoven, or Willie Nelson. It amazes me how these composers' music alters my attitude.

Technology today provides you with an incredible array of equipment so that you can listen to music any time, any place, from listening to music in your car, your office, home, or while you're enjoying fresh air.

Experiment with yourself. When your attitude starts to turn negative, turn on music and test how if affects you. If you feel music changing your attitude, turning from negative to positive, place your radio, tapes, or records near you and when you feel low, instead of reaching for a snack, turn on your music.

Some music inspires, while other music has a calming effect. Relaxing music gives you time to gather your fragmented mental processes together.

Each of you differs in the kind of music you find relaxing. I have a friend who relaxes to acid rock. I can't relax to that, but I can to Handel's Water Music Suite and to singer Phil Collins.

You've probably heard the nature recordings of ocean waves crashing onto the seashore, of the wind blowing in the forest, of rain storms, of loons calling across a lake. These sounds relax your mind. If you like to use music to relax you while you regain control, keep the records or cassettes just as available as the food you used to eat to calm yourself.

Books

Books can open windows to your mind. This may sound corny, but motivational books can alter your moods. Even books of quotations can elevate your mood. That's why I used quotations in this book. Quotations inspire me.

Quotations are condensations of the wisdom of people experienced in life. Poetry can do this. Who can read Rudyard Kipling's *If* and not feel inspired?

Norman Vincent Peale and Og Mandino, the most successful inspirational writers and speakers in the United States, write inspirational books. The content in these books has inspired millions of readers.

The Bible serves as another book of inspiration. The Sermon on the Mount admonishes people to take one day at a time. This is particularly important if you need to lose 100 or more pounds and lack inspiration.

You can inspire yourself by reading biographies of great leaders in politics, medicine, business, or athletics.

Many readers find that action/adventure and mystery novels, books with fast-moving plots, give their mental processes a chance to rest, to regenerate after stressful experiences. Numerous American presidents, including President Kennedy, read mystery, adventure, and, yes, just good trashy novels with their exaggerated characters and plot.

Friends

Cultivate acquaintances and friendships with enthusiastic people. Some people stay more on the positive side, or enthusiastic side, all the time. Their mood infects others and instills humor, enthusiasm, and a positive sense of achievement.

In part, you must look for these individuals in your life. Let me give you an example.

John, one of my patients, had a great number of medical problems. If he had chosen, he could have been despondent all the time. When John came into my office, or I saw him in the hospital, he always made me smile, no matter in what mood I had been. When we parted each time, I felt good.

John had that special gift of imbuing others with happiness. He seemed to emit, or give off, a positive energy. Anyone who came in contact with him benefitted from him.

The nurses in the hospital loved to tend to John's medical needs. He always made them feel good. When I asked him how he felt, he always answered, "Great!" He actually behaved as if he felt great.

I believe that John lived ten years longer than his medical conditions should have allowed. Yes, cancer had spread throughout his body, he had heart disease, and so many serious diseases. John taught me, the nurses, and other hospital personnel about positive living.

Despite your circumstances, you can have a positive attitude.

Unfortunately, some people give off a negative energy. You must avoid these people when you diet.

Once you achieve a positive image of yourself and have given it a chance to take root, you can, with greater assurance, associate with negative people.

What do you do if that negative individual is your spouse? This makes dieting difficult, but not impossible. At the least, I hope you can inspire your spouse to read this book so that individual can understand you and your goals.

Sit down with that person and explain your goals. If this

doesn't work, you must develop a deaf ear to their comments. Your health is worth the effort.

If this makes you feel any better, I've seen this problem over and over again. A spouse goes on an Ultrafit Diet program and starts to feel and look better. Soon, the negative spouse wants to participate in the Ultrafit Diet program. I can't promise you such a happy ending all the time, so prepare yourself to continue your program despite this obstacle.

Diet

I saved the best for last. Diet influences your emotions. I believe that swings in your blood sugar and amino acid levels influence your mood.

The Ultrafit Diets, with their multiple feedings, lead to a constant blood sugar and amino acid level. This constant level staves off lethargy in the afternoon. It sustains your thinking capacity.

Think about the last time you ate a large meal loaded with fatty foods and sugars. If you ate that meal late in the evening, you probably didn't sleep well. If you ate it at midday, you probably got very sleepy in the afternoon.

Lethargy makes you vulnerable to depression and guilt. You can hold these monsters at bay with any of the Ultrafit Diets.

Visualization

What your mind can conceive, your body will achieve. If you decide to conquer and gain permanent control over your weight, you must visualize yourself as thin. For *permanent* weight loss, I believe visualization holds the key.

How many times have you lost unsightly pounds only to look in the mirror and still see yourself as fat? If you see yourself as fat, even as the scales and skin calipers tell you that you weigh your ideal weight, you suffer from a body image problem.

You've seen yourself fat for so long that your mind conceives of you as being fat. I believe that many people regain weight because they become discouraged when they constantly see themselves as fat.

Sylvia had this problem. Sylvia weighed 178 pounds and stood five feet, five inches when she started on the Ultrafit Diet. Eight months later, when she came into my office for a checkup and to be weighed, she asked me a very important question.

"Doctor," she said, "not only have I lost 60 pounds, I've gone from a size 16 to size 8 dress. Why, when I look in the mirror, do I see size 16 when I know better?"

I knew I had to help Sylvia immediately or she would start to regain her weight. I'd seen this happen before.

"Sylvia, you have a body image problem," I told her. "Imagine your brain as a photographic film. You imprinted the pictures it holds by having looked in the mirror all these years.

"Think back. You started gaining weight with the birth of your child twelve years ago. That picture resembles an old picture album that you've looked at for years. It's going to take practice to change the picture you've imprinted on your mind."

Sylvia had lost weight, but she had not achieved long-term weight control. I instructed Sylvia in mental homework. I told her this homework became just as necessary as her maintenance diet if she wanted to achieve permanent weight loss.

I told her to practice her homework three times a day—in the morning when she arose, at lunch, and at bedtime just before she went to sleep. Here's what I told Sylvia.

—Close your eyes and picture yourself as thin.
—Visualize how you look to others, not just yourself.
—Ask your husband what he sees.

—Have someone photograph you now. Compare this photograph with one taken when you weighed 178 pounds.

—Study the pictures for one month, and then destroy the picture of yourself at 178 pounds.

—Give away all your size 16 clothes.

You and Sylvia must get rid of the old images and replace them with new images. My efforts focused on helping Sylvia believe what she had accomplished. Sylvia managed to believe her new image after six months.

You must do this, too. Make yourself believe what you actually weigh when you reach your ideal weight.

You must weigh yourself every day until you convince yourself that you look slender. When you find your weight climbing more than five pounds above your ideal weight, go back on the Ultrafit Reducing Diet or the Amino Acid Diet until you reestablish your goal weight.

You must do this constant external checking until you establish the new image of yourself in your mind. At this point, your automatic pilot takes over and you need to check your bathroom scales only once a week and your percent body fat once a month. This keeps you mentally honest with yourself.

An Image Disease

Anorexia nervosa offers an extreme example of the negative photographic image that some people have of themselves. I follow a few patients with this disorder.

People with this disease have a total inability to see themselves as they actually are. Even when these people reach a skeletal state, they still see themselves as fat. If asked to draw a picture of themselves, they draw fat people.

One of the cornerstones of therapy involves helping such people to see themselves as they really are.

Athlete Techniques

Arnold Schwarzenegger, in his book *Education of a Body-builder*, discusses his personal experience with visualization. In his case, he idolized another bodybuilder, Reg Park. Arnold actually cut out pictures of Reg and placed them in places where he saw them frequently. This helped him visualize the shape he wanted to attain.

Over the next few years, Arnold's body actually took on many of the same structural characteristics of Reg's. Arnold did not stop there. When he exercised, he visualized his biceps becoming as big as a mountain.

World-class athletes use positive imagery. They develop the ability to visualize themselves achieving record-breaking levels. They repeat the image over and over until it becomes a reality of the mind.

Carl Lewis, a world-class sprinter and broad jumper, used this technique before he broke several world records.

Set Goals

Visualization techniques require that you set goals. Body-building has taught me that goal setting becomes important if I plan to progress and maintain my enthusiasm. You must set goals. You want to establish long-term goals. Decide what you want to weigh, and how you want to look at that weight. In between, set intermediate goals. Do simple things, such as deciding to take your belt up a notch, wear a dress that you haven't been able to fit in for years. Visualize yourself in that suit or dress.

If you are a woman, buy yourself a new dress and hang it in your closet so that you can see it twice a day. Visualize yourself fitting into that dress and how good you will look wearing it.

If you are a man, do the same as a woman. Buy that new suit and hang it in the closet where you must look at it twice a day so that you can visualize yourself fitting into it.

Repeat. Repeat

Use repetition in the next phase of your visualization plan. Each time you eat a meal on your Ultrafit Diet plan, repeat this process. Actively visualize your muscle and your mitochondria burning your fuel and excess fat, and giving you plenty of energy.

This is not a dumb idea. Repeat the visualization five or six times a day, each time you eat. The repetition makes the process part of your unconscious mind and allows you to think of yourself in a totally new way.

You can learn this behavior. Visualization is a learned skill, just as you learn management skills, accounting, medical, or carpentry skills. The more you practice it, the more effective you become in shaping images.

You can take advantage of this technique to help you achieve the Ultrafit State.

Stress Eating

Imagine this scene. It's four o'clock in the afternoon and you're in the house trying to straighten up your teenage son's room for the tenth time. The telephone rings.

It's Mrs. Adams, your fourth-grader's teacher. She wants you to come in for a teacher-parent conference. It seems your child talks too much during social studies. In addition, he started two fights in the hall. You feel stressed.

While you contemplate how to discipline your children, you unconsciously reach for a bag of chips and start to nibble. You just started stress eating.

You're not hungry, but eating under these circumstances makes you feel better. Why?

Doctors don't know exactly but believe that the act of eating produces a group of hormones that serve as a natural tranquilizer for your overworked nervous system. In fact, these hormones, known as endorphins, are the same hormones produced when you exercise and they have the same tranquilizing effect.

Individuals react differently to stress, just as do animals. When scientists put laboratory animals under stress, for example, subjecting rabbits to cold, and give them free access to food, some eat more, some stop eating. Humans subjected to stress do the same thing.

In the laboratory, approximately 60 percent of a random group of people responded to stress with an increased caloric intake.

You should know this important health fact about yourself. You should know whether you eat under stress. Much stress eating takes place at an unconscious level. "The devil made me do it" may contain more truth than most of us know.

The unconscious nature that stimulates much of stress eating makes it more difficult to control. You must control stress eating if you intend to achieve long-term weight control.

Consider the case of Sue Ann. At 29 years of age, Sue Ann came to me because she didn't like her appearance. She weighed 165 pounds and stood five feet, four inches. Up until this point, she had no health problems.

I put her on the Ultrafit Reducing Diet, which she followed closely. After eight weeks, Sue Ann had lost only three pounds. She showed me her diet records, which she kept daily.

I sensed that Sue Ann told me the truth when she said she ate nothing not listed on her records. I believed her. We began to talk about her family and her relationships.

I learned that she had a preoccupied and emotionally distant husband who did not help her with the behavior of their bright but difficult five-year-old son. She felt frustrated at her husband's lack of attention and her own inability to fulfill her role as a mother.

We decided she should continue to follow the Ultrafit Reducing Diet until we unlocked the mystery to her lack of weight loss. One evening, while I worked late at the office, I received a telephone call from Sue Ann.

"Doc," she said with excitement, "I know the answer. Tonight while I cooked supper, my husband said, 'Is fried catfish on your diet?'

" 'Of course not,' I told him. 'Why are you eating it now?' he said.

"I hate catfish, Doc. I can't stand to eat it fixed any way. Yet I had my mouth full and I didn't even know it."

Armed with this awareness, we began to deal with Sue Ann's unconscious eating. Every time she became unable to deal with her son's trying behavior, or her husband's lack of attention, she ate any food close at hand.

Sue Ann had a good mental eraser, one of the few I've known. I began to work with Sue Ann, teaching her positive ways to deal with stress. I enlisted the help of her husband and asked him to follow the Ultrafit Maintenance Diet while she followed the Reducing Diet.

In three months, Sue Ann had lost 32 pounds. Her husband not only showed a renewed emotional and physical interest in her, he started to help her with the day-to-day problems of their son.

The important message from this story? You must take a personal inventory of your eating behavior. You must be rigidly honest with yourself in this evaluation. You should enlist the help of those close to you in this analysis.

Although I do not believe unconscious eating represents a major cause of obesity in this country, Sue Ann's experience indicates it can be an important cause.

What do you do if you discover you eat under stress? You can't avoid all stress. You shouldn't even try. Stress, if directed positively, can prepare you to perform well whether at home or the office. It can focus your thinking and turn up your energy level.

Without stress, you could develop a boring life. I believe that more people overeat from boredom than stress. Boredom can precipitate negative stress.

Coping with Stress

To cope with stress, learn the source of stress. Then use one of the coping skills outlined earlier in Chapter 6 to help you rework your attitude.

I have a friend who is a stress eater and who enjoys mowing her lawn. During one particularly hectic period of her life, she mowed her lawn every day. The neighbors thought her somewhat strange, but she worked her way through her problems and kept her weight and her emotional well-being intact.

I think you will agree that her method of handling stress beat the two-beers-and-a-bag-of-potato-chips approach to life's problems that I've seen all too often.

Let me teach you coping skills that help you regain control. I saw an anonymous quote not long ago that serenity is not freedom from the storm but calm amidst the storm. Let me repeat: You cannot nor should you try to avoid all stress.

The suggestions I offer include activities listed under the heads "Exercise," "Music," "Books," "Friends," and "Visualization." Activities suggested represent only a few ideas to help you regain control of your life.

Try Using Quiet Time

A gap stretches between your arrival home and supper. Stress eaters tend to fill this gap with munching. This holds particularly true for working mothers who must prepare supper for a demanding family.

In this case, I recommend a small ritual for my patients to follow. Sit down, I tell them. Put your feet up for ten minutes after you arrive home. During this time, listen to some pleasing music. Or daydream.

Quiet time gives you the amazing ability to help you renew your sense of self-control. What you actually do during the ten minutes isn't as important as giving yourself the time to reestablish control over your nervous system.

New Ways to Show Love

Food belongs in our rituals in life. From the time we're born, we associate mother's love with food. Mothers show members of their families love by food offerings. Eating becomes a way of expressing love for your family, especially your extended family of children and relatives.

Eating becomes a social event to establish the pecking order in life. Business colleagues show respect by taking associates to restaurants that offer fine dining. Friends invite each other into their homes. We measure each other by how well we feed one another.

For centuries, a person's ability to set a good meal before friends offered one of the most important ways a person could demonstrate to his friends his position in life. Our consumption of this food became one of the unfortunate ways we showed our respect and appreciation for this position.

How many of you, when asked to a friend's home, can say no when offered a piece of cake or pie? Why? You feel pressured not to insult your host or hostess. You have succumbed to the social pressures of eating.

As a businessman or -woman, you want to impress your client by taking him or her to a fine restaurant. The client, who does not want to insult you by refusing your offer, crumbles to the social pressure of eating.

The social pressures of eating go back generations when food scarcity presented serious problems. Today, the abundance of food presents a different problem. We don't need to eliminate the rituals we develop around food and eating. We just need to create new ways of eating.

I suggest to mothers that they show love by offering their children snacks of raw and dried fruits, raw vegetables such as carrots and celery, and bread, rice cakes, whole grain cereals. To satisfy the child with a sweet tooth, nothing beats the sweets like dates, raisins, and figs.

You can literally love your children to death by giving

them fried chicken, fried potatoes, and chocolate pie. Offer the chicken baked, the potatoes steamed and seasoned with herbs, and for dessert a fruit salad made with fresh fruit or mixed in jello. Nature offers a limited number of sweets, and most are found in fruits.

A new kind of restaurant today makes eating out less a problem when you eat the Ultrafit way. The next time you take a business client to a restaurant, try one that offers nouvelle cuisine, the newest cooking style. Some of these restaurants specialize in foods that contain little or no fat.

Better restaurants encourage diners to speak to the chef before arriving and request specially prepared meals. The same restaurants like for diners to talk with their waiter and request that the chef not use fat in the preparation, whether the food happens to be Chinese, Italian, French, or home-cooked.

Show respect for your business client by demonstrating your concern for her or his health. In today's business environment, it's acceptable to suggest to your host or hostess that you prefer to eat at a restaurant that offers low-fat food preparation. The topic of health offers a comfortable conversational subject to start any business discussion. You might find it surprising how many of your colleagues know about cholesterol levels and percent body fat.

Women who stay at home have just as great a problem as business people in resisting the social pressure of overeating or eating fat-laden foods. Virginia, one of my overweight patients, belongs to a bridge group that plays four days a week. Virginia needed to lose 60 pounds.

"Doctor," Virginia pleaded, "what am I going to do? When I go to my friends' homes, they always have dessert ready. How can I not hurt their feelings by refusing to eat their food?"

"You've got to set the example, Virginia," I told her. "The next time you hostess the bridge group, serve freshly baked bread, without butter, as your love offering."

Virginia's experience started a new topic of conversation about health and nutrition. Members of her bridge group asked for her bread recipe made with five kinds of flours and grains. Other bridge friends began to experiment with recipes that offered originality while fitting into the Ultrafit way of eating.

Remember. You must take charge of your health. No one benefits more than you when you determine what you put into your body.

Two of the most sophisticated people I know, a couple who lived in France and England, always serve their guests elegant meals low in fat. They always serve a wide variety of fruits for dessert. They arrange the fruits on the plate in such a way that their guests look forward to seeing the artful array.

Grandmothers have a particular problem. Helen, a grandmother who is one of my patients, has major medical problems, all related to her obesity and her elevated cholesterol. Her grandchildren have become her stumbling block to solving her health problems.

Helen has four children and eight grandchildren. One or more grandchildren spends weekends at Helen's home during the school year. Helen feels compelled to keep the cookie jar filled, just as her grandmother did for her. Helen can't resist the temptation to sample the cookies with her grandchildren.

As a fellow cookie-holic, I sympathized with Helen. I told her how I had overcome my cookie-eating problem with the pig-out meal. I suggested that she, too, try eliminating cookies from her home. She could show love by serving her grandchildren the fruits, vegetables, bread, rice cakes, cereals, all kinds of healthful foods that offer rich sources of vitamins and minerals, if she set her mind to working.

Check Your PMA

Check your PMA, your Positive Mental Attitude. Too many people stumble out of bed and feel their way into the day without determining their mental state.

> You have to study a great deal to know a little.
> —BARON DE MONTESQUIEU

CHAPTER TWELVE

Vitamins, Minerals, and Water vs Free Radicals

You can reach the Ultrafit State without knowing anything about vitamins, minerals, water, or free radicals. If you plan to make the Ultrafit State a part of your life, I believe you must understand your body and what happens to the food you eat.

I told you that you could eat the correct amounts of foods in the Ultrafit Amino Acid, Reducing, and Maintenance Diets without stopping to determine the grams of fat, protein, and carbohydrate your body required. Remember that I said, too, that if you planned to learn to eat a new way, you had to understand your specific body requirements. I've provided you with a chart at the end of this chapter that gives the exact amounts of the different vitamins and minerals you need.

Now, I'm asking you to better understand your body chemistry. I'm asking you to understand that chemicals make up all food. Protein, fat, and carbohydrates provide some of those chemicals that comprise food. However, that's not the whole story. Your body requires specific amounts of vitamins, minerals, and water to help you achieve the ultimate state of health, the Ultrafit State.

As your body uses these chemicals taken from foods, your body makes a byproduct called free radicals.

Free Radicals

Every day, each of us produces millions of free radicals, compounds that have one unpaired electron in their atomic makeup. Free radicals result from the chemical breakdown of foodstuff.

Even if you try, you cannot escape free radicals. They appear in your body and the atmosphere. However, your body produces substances that keep them from getting out of control.

Uncontrolled free radicals damage proteins, fats, and nucleic acids, your DNA that contains your genetic blueprint. The damage results in DNA mutations, which lead to cancer and the aging process of senility. Free radical-damaged DNA also leads to arthritis, hardening of the arteries, and the declining function of your immune system as you age.

What do free radicals have to do with the Ultrafit Way of Life? The more fat you carry on your body, the more fat you take in in your diet, the more free radicals you produce.

In addition to fat, ionizing radiation, such as sunlight, produces free radicals. That's one of the reasons we doctors warn people to avoid excessive sunlight.

Since you cannot avoid these radicals, what can you do to reduce the risk?

Avoid excess fat in your diet.

Avoid excess sunlight. That means no sunburns.

Avoid excess alcohol.

Avoid cigarette smoke.

Avoid automobile fumes.

In addition to living in moderation and striving to live in a clean environment, you can enhance your diet. You must make sure that you consume adequate amounts of vitamins A, C, E, and the minerals zinc and selenium. Each of these play an important role in protecting your body against free radicals.

Certain vitamins help to protect you against the ill effects that free radicals cause in your body.

When you understand vitamins, minerals, and water and their effects, you can better protect yourself against your enemy, free radicals.

Vitamin/Mineral Controversy

Every day patients come to me saying, "Doc, you know something about nutrition. Should I take vitamin supplements?"

That question tells me something you and I know. Medical research has not written the final chapter on the body's need for and use of vitamins. Controversy surrounds how much of a particular vitamin or mineral your body needs, because we're still learning about the role of vitamins and minerals in the body's chemistry.

However, we do know certain facts. The Research Council of the National Academy of Sciences makes specific recommendations, based on medical research, that adults and children consume certain amounts of vitamins and minerals each day. You will find these recommendations in the chart at the end of this chapter.

Doctors know that if you do not consume the recommended amounts you will develop diseases from deficiencies. We know, too, that if you consume too much, you develop toxic diseases.

Why the controversy, then, if a scientific body provides you a guideline? Research continues to reveal new information about how the body uses vitamins and minerals. I'm sure you read these findings in your newspapers and magazines.

Many doctors and nutritionists do not recommend that you take vitamin or mineral supplements if you eat a balanced diet.

Having said that, let me describe a controversy around that recommendation. In a study done in the state of Washington, a survey of dietitians and nutritionists revealed that 80 percent of those surveyed did not recommend that anyone who ate a balanced diet should take vitamin/mineral supplements. Yet, 60 percent of all those surveyed took vitamin/mineral supplements on a regular basis themselves. You can see that what people say and what they do are sometimes two different things.

Here's what I recommend. If you follow the Ultrafit Maintenance Diet, consume more than 1500 calories each day, and do not have special body needs, you do not need vitamin pills for general good health. The Ultrafit Maintenance Diet provides your body with all the vitamins it needs. That's why you feel so good and have so much energy.

You do, however, need to take a calcium and iron supplement to prevent a deficiency state. You need to take a product that gives you 1000 milligrams of calcium a day. You need to select a separate product that gives you 14 milligrams of iron a day.

If you eat less than 1200 calories a day, you do need to take a vitamin/mineral supplement. For example, if you follow the Amino Acid Ultrafit Diet or the 1000-calorie Ultrafit Reducing Diet, you need to take a vitamin/mineral supplement. I'm not going to get into naming commercial products, simply because you have available to you a bewildering array of very good products.

Here's what I do suggest.

Look at the chart at the end of this chapter. Take the chart with you to the store and select a product that provides you with the quantities listed as your daily requirements.

I do believe, personally, that certain vitamins and minerals act as health enhancers. These include vitamins C and E and the mineral selenium. I believe they provide my body cells with a margin of safety against disease, particularly those diseases such as cancer and hardening of the arteries associated with free radicals. I do take 2000 milligrams of vitamin C, 400 units of vitamin E, and 100 micrograms of selenium a day.

Vitamins

In my medical practice, I find some patients believe vitamins mean One-A-Day. Others think vitamins relate to B vitamins that give you energy and make you hungry. Still others associate vitamins with vitamin C and colds.

All of these beliefs contain elements of truth. They are not the whole truth.

That's the problem with vitamins. Facts get mixed with opinions that get mixed with beliefs that get mixed with myth.

Let me try to set you straight.

1. Vitamins are organic compounds, as opposed to inorganic compounds such as minerals.
2. Your body requires vitamins for normal body metabolism.
3. Your body cannot make vitamins.
4. All unprocessed food contains vitamins.
5. A deficiency of a specific vitamin results in a specific disease.
6. Vitamins act as aids to enzymes and co-enzymes in the chemical reactions in your body.
7. Vitamins fall into two broad categories: water-soluble and fat-soluble.

To teach you a little more about vitamins, I am going to discuss both water-soluble and fat-soluble vitamins in some detail.

Water-Soluble Vitamins

Water-soluble vitamins include vitamin C and the B vitamins. Water-soluble means that the vitamin readily dissolves in water. Your body will eliminate excess amounts of these vitamins in your urine. That's why your urine takes on a different odor when you take large amounts of B vitamins, particularly riboflavin—B_2.

Science recognizes eight B vitamins as essential to your health. Don't become confused by the numbering system science has given various B vitamins. Researchers gave these vitamins their names and numbers as the vitamins were discovered. Some go by numbers, others by names.

In your quest to understand your body chemistry of vitamins, let me tell you how each of the essential B vitamins works and what happens when you develop a deficiency or consume too much.

Thiamine—B_1 ENERGY

Your body needs thiamine for the final metabolism and use of carbohydrates and most amino acids. Thiamine becomes extremely important in building proteins, which include your muscles, and in burning carbohydrate fuels. That's how the B vitamins got their reputation for giving you energy.

Thiamine deficiency produces problems in a wide variety of organs, including your brain and peripheral nerves, your heart and skeletal muscles, and your gastrointestinal tract. A deficiency results in weakened and atrophied muscles, and in swelling in these tissues. This disease condition is known as beriberi.

In the United States, doctors most commonly see this deficiency in people who drink too much alcohol. How much is too much alcohol? If you drink more than one and a half ounces of alcohol a day, the excess alcohol accumulates in your body because your body cannot metabolize this much alcohol. The alcohol interferes with thiamine's chemical reactions.

Tingling and burning in your hands and feet give you the first symptoms of deficiency. As the deficiency progresses, congestive heart failure develops as the heart muscle weakens and the heart can no longer pump blood. The foods that supply abundant amounts of thiamine include whole wheat and oatmeal cereals and breads, peas, pasta, dry beans, and asparagus.

Niacin or Nicotinic Acid—B_3

Niacin acts directly to utilize carbohydrates. The enzymes it works with operate in all cells of the body. A deficiency produces a disease called pellagra. This disease involves the brain, skin, and gastrointestinal tract.

Scientists discovered this vitamin during the Depression when poor people ate diets made up almost exclusively of corn, a food that doesn't contain the amount of niacin your body needs. Doctors still see this vitamin deficiency, again, in individuals who drink too much alcohol.

Doctors use niacin as a drug today in the treatment of elevated cholesterol. Large doses of niacin dilate the small arteries, which can cause flushing and itching. When people who take niacin develop flushed skin and itching, it does not mean that they have an allergic reaction; it's simply a normal side effect. Some ear, nose, and throat specialists use niacin to dilate the arteries in the inner ear in persons who have ringing in their ears.

Among the foods that can supply your body needs are whole grain breads and cereals, chicken breast, fish, and eggs.

Riboflavin—B_2

Riboflavin aids your metabolism of carbohydrates. A riboflavin deficiency produces some of the same problems as a niacin deficiency. This happens in people who eat highly refined foods and almost no fresh fruits and vegetables. Doctors see mild cases of riboflavin deficiency. In my practice, I usually spot this deficiency in a person who's developed cracks in the corner of his mouth.

The deficiency causes gastrointestinal upset, burning of your skin and eyes, cracking and scaling in the corners of your mouth, headaches, mental depression, forgetfulness, and symptoms related to your muscle strength and function.

Green leafy vegetables, eggs, milk, broccoli, and asparagus provide good sources of riboflavin.

Vitamin B$_{12}$ *ENERGY / GOOD MEMORY*

Most of you have heard of this vitamin. It enjoys the reputation of being the supreme energy vitamin. It functions as a co-enzyme to make red blood cells, and acts in the brain and peripheral nerves to maintain their proper transmission of nerve impulses. Your body uses vitamin B$_{12}$ to reproduce DNA within the cell.

Doctors also see this deficiency in patients who have pernicious anemia. We see the deficiency, too, in patients with tingling and burning of the hands and feet, and in elderly people with memory loss or dementia.

Dairy products, eggs, meat, fish, or poultry provide your body's need for this vitamin. Because B$_{12}$ only exists in animal products, strict vegetarians, who do not eat these foods, must take supplements of this vitamin.

Folic Acid

Like vitamin B$_{12}$, your body uses folic acid to reproduce DNA within the cell. Your body also needs folic acid to produce red blood cells. A deficiency results in anemia.

I see this deficiency in alcoholics and in people with seizure disorders who take Dilantin, a drug used to control seizures. (Dilantin interferes with the absorption of folic acid.)

Pregnant women and nursing mothers need supplemental

amounts of this vitamin to ensure proper development of the fetus. Women who take birth control pills need extra amounts of this vitamin because the birth control pills interfere with folic acid's chemical reactions in the liver.

Green leafy vegetables and whole grain cereals and breads offer abundant supplies of folic acid.

Pyridoxine—Vitamin B_6

Scientists call vitamin B_6 the protein vitamin. It serves in the manufacture of certain amino acids and to transport amino acids across cell membranes.

If you take this vitamin in large amounts for several weeks, you can develop peripheral neuropathy, a disease of the nerves that prevents your nerves from transmitting proper signals. People with this disorder develop numbness in their hands and feet.

Skin diseases can result from a deficiency.

Doctors use vitamin B_6 to treat carpal tunnel syndrome, a swelling of the nerve at your wrist. We use it, too, in women who develop PMS or premenstrual syndrome—bloating, abdominal pain, headaches, depression, and weight gain immediately prior to their menstrual periods. Wheat and corn products, poultry, fish, and bananas are good sources.

Pantothenic Acid

You need this B vitamin to protect you from the effects of free radicals. No researcher has described in scientific literature the effects of a deficiency in humans. Laboratory animals deprived of this vitamin demonstrate stunted growth, reproduction failure, and graying hair.

All unrefined foods contain adequate amounts of this vitamin. Whole grain breads and cereals and milk are good sources.

Biotin

It is not common to have a deficiency of biotin, the eighth B vitamin, because your intestinal tract bacteria make it. Your body sponges off this supply.

You can develop a deficiency, however, if you take large amounts of oral antibiotics while, at the same time, you consume less than 500 calories a day. Perhaps you've read the admonition not to eat large amounts of raw egg white. That's because raw egg white binds biotin and prevents your body from absorbing it.

Whole grain cereals and breads and yeast offer good sources of biotin.

Vitamin C

The Ultrafit Diets provide such a rich supply of citrus fruits and dark green vegetables, sources of vitamin C, that I never worry about you getting scurvy, the disease that results from not enough vitamin C.

I do believe that supplemental doses of vitamin C boost your immune power and protect you against free radicals. In other words, your wounds heal faster, your colds and virus infections last a shorter period of time, and you become less apt to develop cancer.

Let me caution you before you get carried away taking too much vitamin C. Large amounts, up to 10 grams or 10000 milligrams a day, cause your urine to become very acidic. When this happens, you run the risk of developing uric acid kidney stones.

Doctors see vitamin C deficiency, or scurvy, primarily in chronic alcoholics. These people develop small hemorrhages in the hair follicles on their legs and arms; their gums bleed; they bleed from their gastrointestinal tract.

Surgeons see delayed wound healing in patients who cannot eat after surgery and thus don't get enough vitamin C.

Fat-Soluble Vitamins

Fat-soluble vitamins dissolve in fat. They include vitamins A, D, E, and K. You know that the Ultrafit Diets provide only small amounts of fat in your diet. Does that mean you can develop a fat-soluble vitamin deficiency if you follow these diets? No, except for the Ultrafit Amino Acid Diet that eliminates fat from your diet. I recommend you add vitamin supplements to your Amino Acid Diet.

Your body requires a minute amount of fat in which to provide the fat necessary for these vitamins to be absorbed. Your body stores fat-soluble vitamins in your liver and other fatty tissues. You can get too much vitamin A and D and develop diseases related to their excess.

Let me take you through the fat-soluble vitamins.

Vitamin A

Your eyes need vitamin A, which helps provide pigmentation for your eyes. If you don't get enough vitamin A, you develop night blindness.

Vitamin A deficiency can produce scaly skin and acne. Sometimes we call this vitamin the anti-infection vitamin because in experiments, animals deprived of vitamin A developed infections in their eyes, kidneys, and respiratory tracts.

A growing body of scientific literature suggests that vitamin A functions as a scavenger for free radicals produced by such things as smoking, air pollution, excessive fat ingestion, or excessive alcohol intake.

Doctors recommend that you do not take more than 5000 units per day. If you take more than 25000 units a day, you can develop dry and scaly skin, increased pressure on your brain, nausea, and vomiting.

This vitamin does not appear in fruits and vegetables, but its precursor vitamin does in green and yellow vegetables and fruits, eggs, and fish. Your body must convert the pre-cursor vitamin to vitamin A, and it does this easily.

Vitamin D

This vitamin increases calcium absorption from your in-testinal tract and helps control your bone formation.

Children who do not get enough vitamin D develop a disease called rickets, a disease of the bone in which the bones get weak and break easily.

Adults with vitamin D deficiency develop a bone disease called osteomalacia, a condition that produces soft bone that fractures easily. Doctors see osteomalacia in the elderly, particularly people who live in colder climates and who do not get much exposure to sunlight.

Doctors use vitamin D, with calcium supplements, to treat another bone disease called osteoporosis, a thinning of the bones that causes them to break easily.

If you consume more than 800 units of vitamin D a day, you can develop problems associated with toxic poisoning. Symptoms include nausea and vomiting and mental depres-sion as your blood calcium level rises too high.

You find vitamin D in dairy products, especially in milk, and in fish such as salmon and sardines. When you expose your body to sunlight, the sun's rays convert a precursor vitamin in your skin to produce vitamin D.

Vitamin E take less than 500 units a day

Scientific researchers still debate how the body uses vi-tamin E because it's hard to induce a human deficiency of this vitamin. In animal experiments, a deficiency causes red blood cell rupture.

You could call this vitamin controversial. Why? It involves the reproductive system in animals. Any time you start talk-ing about sex, you cause controversy.

Doctors do use vitamin E as a drug. Some use it to treat patients with hardening of the arteries. In doses up to 800 units a day, it has anti-blood-clotting properties. Doctors use it in doses of 400 to 800 units a day to treat fibrocystic disease of the breast, an extremely common, benign yet painful condition in women.

Vitamin E acts as an antioxidant that destroys free radicals. In cell culture, grown in the laboratory, vitamin E decreases damage done to DNA by cigarette smoke. These studies prompted doctors to use doses of vitamin E in people who smoke cigarettes and/or are exposed to large amounts of ozone found in high smog areas. Vitamin E aids in the proper function of your muscles, especially your mitochondria, which we now know burn your excess fat.

Do not take excessive amounts of vitamin E. What's excessive? If you consume more than 800 units a day for several weeks, you run the risk of developing a peculiar condition of the muscle in which their membranes rupture.

Good food sources of vitamin E include wheat germ and whole wheat grains and cereals.

Vitamin K

The bacteria in your gastrointestinal tract make this vitamin for you. Normal healthy individuals cannot possibly develop a deficiency in vitamin K. However, if you take antibiotics, either orally or through your veins, for a long period of time, you can become deficient in this vitamin.

Vitamin K helps your liver make blood-clotting factors. When you become deficient, your blood will not clot easily. You can develop a pseudo deficiency if you take Coumadin, a drug used to treat heart disease and strokes.

Minerals

Minerals, like vitamins, act as co-enzymes to help chemical reactions take place in your body. In addition, minerals act as building blocks for your bones, teeth, hair, and nails.

While the structure of vitamins can be quite complex, minerals are more simple in structure. Minerals exist in nature in rocks and soil. You can literally dig minerals out of rocks.

You can develop diseases from mineral deficiencies, just as you can from vitamin deficiencies. You can suffer mineral toxic states from too much intake, too.

Over and over, medical studies show that more people in this country suffer from calcium and iron deficiencies than any other deficiency. My medical experience confirms these studies.

Calcium use Calcium citrate

Even television commercials tell you that you need calcium for your bones and teeth. Your muscle contractions, including your heart muscle function, and your nervous system, which includes your brain and peripheral nerves, must have adequate amounts of calcium to function properly.

An estimated 60 percent of adults and 80 percent of teenagers do not take in the recommended amounts of calcium. Calcium deficiency is the most common of all deficiencies.

Osteoporosis with thinning of the bones, rheumatoid arthritis with accelerated destruction of the joints, and degenerative arthritis all result from calcium deficiency. Medical research now focuses on using calcium as a drug to prevent colon cancer in certain individuals at high risk. Doctors also use it to treat high blood pressure in certain individuals.

Can you consume too much calcium? Sure you can. You can develop kidney stones from taking too much calcium, and by taking the wrong kind of calcium supplements. Most calcium supplements consist of calcium carbonate, the end product of limestone or oyster shells. Some people cannot metabolize calcium carbonate and their bodies turn it into kidney stones. These people must take calcium supplements made from calcium citrate. The citrate found in this compound inhibits kidney stone formation.

Dairy products provide the main source of calcium in food.

Certain green vegetables do contain calcium, but they are not as practical a source.

Phosphorus

Phosphorus interacts in almost every chemical reaction in your body. It acts as a co-enzyme. It works with calcium to form bone. It gets involved in the formation of ATP (adenosine triphosphate), the major energy storehouse of the body.

Can you get a deficiency of phosphorus? Yes, but not easily. Phosphorus appears in all natural foods. You'd literally need to starve yourself to develop a deficiency of this mineral.

Magnesium

Magnesium works as a co-enzyme in your cells, aiding in the burning of carbohydrate. It is involved in the proper function of the central nervous system and aids in muscle contraction. In addition, it interacts with calcium in the formation of bone and teeth.

Doctors see magnesium deficiency in alcoholics and in people who take diuretics because the body eliminates this mineral through the urine. Excessive magnesium can cause muscle paralysis and depression of the central nervous system. Doctors take advantage of magnesium's depressant effect to treat convulsions in pregnant women suffering from eclampsia, a complex toxic medical problem of pregnancy.

Iron

Hemoglobin, the oxygen-carrying pigment of blood, must have iron to function. Iron also works in the energy production system found in the mitochondria.

We see iron deficiency, in the form of anemia, as the second most common deficiency in the United States. Menstruating women in particular suffer from iron deficiency.

Occasionally people develop a toxic disease from taking too much iron. This condition is called hemochromatosis—excess iron in the liver, heart, testicles, and pituitary gland.

Food sources include dark green and leafy vegetables. In truth, beef serves as a source of iron and of many of the vitamins that your body requires; however, I have chosen to list only those foods that belong in the Ultrafit Diets.

Trace Elements

Certain minerals carry the designation of trace elements, that is, minerals that appear in minute amounts in foods and the body. Yet, if you do not get enough of each trace element, you can suffer a deficiency disease. *Iodine* became one of the first trace elements to be recognized. Researchers found that people who did not consume enough developed goiter. The body uses iodine in the formation of the thyroid hormone, which regulates the metabolic rate in all cells.

Iodine deficiency still occurs, but it is rarely seen since you can buy iodine-enriched bread and salt.

I consider *zinc* and *selenium* two other critical trace elements. Zinc plays an integral role in many enzymes. It becomes especially important in the metabolism of carbon dioxide, a toxic byproduct of metabolism in your cells. Zinc also functions in the digestion of protein in the gastrointestinal tract.

If you eat a normal diet, you probably get enough zinc. People who suffer a deficiency usually lose their sense of taste. Doctors use it experimentally as a drug to treat enlargement of the prostate. Doctors use it as a booster to strengthen your immune system. Surgeons use it to help in wound healing.

The trace element selenium acts as a co-enzyme. It works with an enzyme called peroxidase, which protects your body from peroxide, one of the key players in the formation of free radicals.

Water

Water provides the largest single element in your body and diet. It forms an integral part of all the Ultrafit Diets. Why?

Every chemical reaction in your body takes place in water. Your body cannot produce energy or burn calories without water. As you lose weight, you lose water and you must replace that water. Well-hydrated muscles work more efficiently, too.

Water can help you control hunger as well. Water can act to fill your stomach and give you that full feeling. A full stomach sends signals to your satiety center that you do not feel hungry.

You cannot always depend on your thirst signal to tell you that you need to drink water. The thirst center in your brain gradually declines with aging, which makes it more important that you develop a habit of drinking water regularly.

In addition, a high-fat, high-protein, low-carbohydrate diet can produce dehydration. Here's how it works. As you increase your fat and protein intake, your body does an incomplete job of burning the fat. When this happens, your body produces substances called ketone bodies.

Ketone bodies pull water from your tissues as you eliminate the ketones through your urine. You can become dehydrated in the process.

How much water should you drink? I recommend that you drink six to eight glasses of water each day. This should meet the needs of people who weigh between 120 and 180 pounds. You should add one glass of water for each 20 pounds over 180.

Unless you have a medical condition, I do not believe you should spend money on special kinds of water, bottled or unbottled. I consider sports drinks, particularly, a waste of your money. Medical studies show that electrolytes and sugar in sports drinks actually delay absorption of the water you need. In fact, as you adjust to heat, your sweat becomes almost like water and contains almost no salt or electrolytes in it.

I learned this lesson, like so many other lessons, the hard way. When I started working out, I lost as much as eight pounds of water during my bodybuilding sessions. At the end of the workout, and for several hours later, I had problems from extreme fatigue (dehydration) and muscle cramps.

At first I tried to replace the fluid I lost by drinking one of the popular electrolyte sports drinks. My stomach felt full, but I remained fatigued and my muscles still cramped.

I changed my workout routine. I started drinking plain water before my workout, and started sipping it during my workouts. As a result, I lost no more than two pounds during vigorous workouts, and I said good-bye to fatigue and cramps.

Now that you know something about the foods you should eat and the vitamin and mineral supplements you may need, it's time to get some shopping information so that you can be sure you buy the right things.

VITAMINS AND RECOMMENDED DOSAGES

VITAMIN	DAILY DOSAGE	SOME DEFICIENCY RESULTS
A	5000 units	Night blindness, scaly skin, acne
D	400 units	Rickets, osteomalacia, osteoporosis
E	30 units	Red blood cell rupture
C	60 mg	Scurvy
Folic Acid	0.4 mg	Anemia
Niacin (B_3)	15 mg equivalents	Pellagra
Riboflavin (B_2)	1.6 mg	Skin abrasions
Thiamine (B_1)	1.3 mg	Beriberi
Pyridoxine (B_6)	2 mg	Skin disease
Cobalamin (B_{12})	5 mcg	Pernicious anemia
Biotin	300 mcg	None known in man
Pantothenic Acid	10 mcg	None known in man

Dosages are measured in units, in milligrams (mg), and in micrograms (mcg).
Each of these measures are fractions of an ounce. In particular:
1 unit = 3/280,000,000 ounce
1 mg = 1/28,000 ounce
1 mcg = 1/28,000,000 ounce

ESSENTIAL MINERALS AND RECOMMENDED DOSAGES

MINERAL	DAILY DOSAGE	SOME SYMPTOMS OF DEFICIENCY
Calcium	1000–1500 mg	Bone disease
Phosphorus	800 mg	Muscular convulsions
Magnesium	325 mg	Muscular convulsions
Iodine	150 mcg	Goiter
Iron	14 mg	Anemia
Zinc	2 mg	Loss of taste

> The first thing to do in life is to do with purpose
> what one proposes to do.
> —PABLO CASALS

CHAPTER THIRTEEN
The Informed Buyer

In the fifteen years since I began my journey in search of the Ultrafit State, I have changed radically. I developed from a person who had no regard for my personal health to a person who knows that each day I can continually change my life through health.

During these years I became an avid reader of labels on food products, vitamin/mineral products, and amino acid supplements, and of research and medical literature that dealt with nutrition.

I believe that in the next fifteen years you will witness an explosion of information on nutrients, exercise, and attitude as they relate to disease. In the past, too many variables in research techniques and equipment clouded answers wrung from studies on the body.

If you have not learned to read labels, if you have not learned how to evaluate published articles and news stories you read about nutrition and health, if you have not learned to understand labels on vitamin/mineral and food supplement containers, you must begin now. Let me share my approach to reading and evaluating.

I spend most of my food shopping time in the fruits and vegetables section in the grocery store. If you watch grocery shoppers, you probably noticed that most people spend less time in the fruits and vegetables section than in any other.

Start paying attention to your own shopping habits. When

you find yourself spending more time in other sections of the grocery store, start reading your own mental label. Check your grocery basket for foods that belong back on the shelf and not in your body.

When you pick up a packaged item, read the label. If you've never read labels before, start by reading labels on all the packaged foods you buy. Get acquainted with what manufacturers print on labels, and the way it's presented.

Pay particular attention to how much makes one serving. Look at the number of grams of fat, protein, and carbohydrate contained in that serving. Look at the *kind* of fat contained in the food.

Food processors disguise fat on labels in various ways. The following terms mean fat:

hydrogenated vegetable oils
lard
shortening
margarine
butter
palm oil
coconut oil
palm kernel oil

Then pay attention to the type of fat. If you see palm oil, coconut oil, or palm kernel oil on a label, think seriously about whether you want to eat the food in that package. Even food manufacturers have begun to eliminate palm and coconut oils from their cereal products because consumers demanded it.

When you see a label that reads 95 or 97 percent fat-free, know that the percentage generally refers to the total weight. For example, a turkey ham label that reads 97 percent fat-free implies that only 3 percent of the calories come from fat. This may mislead you. That 3 percent refers to the *total weight* of the ham, a ham made up mostly of water. In reality, *a third of the calories come from fat* in a turkey ham.

How many times have you seen "cholesterol-free" margarine or oil? If you read this book, you know that it's the total fat in your diet that counts, not the food's cholesterol content. Food processors use these scare words to imply that it's okay to eat their particular food. Lots of foods that are cholesterol-free are laden with fat.

Food manufacturers get particularly clever about disguising the amount of sugar in a food. Breakfast cereals, especially, contain different kinds of sugars. The following words all mean sugar:

fructose
sucrose
glucose
corn syrup
molasses
honey
dextrose

The more a manufacturer disguises the content of a food, the more you know you want less of that food. For more information on food labeling, you can get a single free copy of the five publications listed below by writing to the Food and Drug Administration, 5600 Fishers Lane, Rockville, Md. 20852.

Metric Measure of Nutrition Labels
Nutrition Labels and the U.S. RDA
Nutrition Labeling—Terms You Should Know
Read the Label, Set a Better Table
The New Look in Food Labels

Vitamin/Mineral Supplements

When you read the label on any food supplement container, compare the list of vitamins/minerals found on the charts in Chapter Twelve. The label should list the specific amount—grams, milligrams, micrograms, units—of each vitamin and/or mineral contained in each tablet. Make sure that the supplement contains *at least* the amounts listed on the Chapter Twelve charts.

The label should also list the percent of the vitamin and/or mineral contained that meets the Recommended Daily Allowance (RDA).

Don't worry about trying to buy supplements that come from natural sources. If you read the label carefully, you will discover that the vitamin/mineral content from "natural" sources comes from manufactured synthetic sources.

Make sure that the vitamin/mineral supplement that you take when you follow the Ultrafit Amino Acid and Ultrafit Reducing Diet contains *no more* than 5000 units of vitamin A, 800 units of vitamin E, 800 units of vitamin D, or 18 mg of iron.

Most vitamin/mineral single-tablet supplements do not contain adequate amounts of calcium or many trace elements. You will need to buy a separate tablet that contains these minerals. Again, make sure the mineral supplement you buy contains the recommended quantities listed in the chart in Chapter Twelve.

For example, make sure you take in at least but not more than 1000 to 1500 milligrams of calcium each day, preferably taken in the form of calcium citrate.

Amino Acid Supplements

When you purchase amino acid supplements, you must read the label carefully to make sure that you receive the amount of amino acids per day contained in 40 to 45 grams of high-quality protein. If the label does not state the grams of protein per serving, you do not want the supplement.

Acceptable predigested proteins are: casein, lactalbumin, egg albumin.

Manufacturers may add certain amino acids to one of the three predigested base proteins in order to enhance its quality. I find this acceptable as long as the amino acids mimic those found in nature.

An ideal amino acid tablet contains these amounts of the essential amino acids:

x 3 =

Lysine	125 mg	375
Arginine	41 mg	123
Histidine	25 mg	75
Typtophan	36 mg	108
Phenylalanine	52 mg	156
Methionine	35 mg	105
Threonine	39 mg	117
Leucine	121 mg	363
Isoleucine	65 mg	195
Valine	70 mg	210

You can purchase predigested amino acid tablets in your local drug or health food stores. Many fitness centers also carry these tablets as do most of the 1,100 branches of General Nutrition Centers (G.N.C.), a national chain of health food stores. Check your Yellow Pages for the location nearest you.

If you prefer mail order, here's a partial list of companies that can provide you with the tablets. I assayed these amino acid tablets to make sure of their adequate protein content. You can depend on these products.

Energen Nutritional Company
14631 Best Ave.
Norwalk, California 90650

Maker's of Kal, Inc.
6415 De Soto Ave.
Woodland Hills, California 91365

Twin Labs
Deer Park
New York, New York 11729

Ultrafit
1326 University Drive
Nacogdoches, Texas 75961

If for some reason you have difficulty obtaining the amino acid or vitamin products recommended in this book, call 1-800-445-0275 for help in locating a source in your area.

	Book per meal	P.D Ameno per TB Cal 34 1/2
Lysine	750	337.6 mg
Arginine	366	353.2 mg
Histidine	150	66 mg
Tryptophan	216	32 mg
Phenylalanine	312	149 mg
Metheonine	210	68 mg
Threonine	234	205.2 mg
Leucine	726	31.0 mg
Isoleucine	290	165.5 mg
Valine	420	195.2 mg

Reading References

To help you become a better consumer, I decided to share some of my best sources.

Arthur C. Guyton, M.D. *Textbook of Medical Physiology*. W. B. Saunders Company, 1986. I consider this the most respected medical text on physiology available. I believe this book belongs on your bookshelf if you want additional information on how your body works.

K. E. Anderson, *et al*. "Nutrient Regulation of Chemical Metabolism in Humans." *Federal Proceedings*, Volume 44, page 130, 1985. This article can give you a more detailed description of how your body processes foodstuffs.

G. A. Bray and D. A. York. "Hypothalamic and Genetic Obesity in Experimental Animals: An Autonomic and Endocrine Hypothesis." *Physiological Review*, Volume 59, page 719, 1979. This article presents some interesting ideas that may help to explain our feeding behavior.

M. F. W. Festing. *Animal Models of Obesity*. Oxford University Press, 1979. This book describes animal models of obesity and has a detailed discussion of the genetics involved.

D. M. Matthews. "Intestinal Absorption of Amino Acids and Peptides." *Proceedings of Nutritional Society*, Volume 31, page 171, 1972. I should warn you that this article gets technical. I've included it in case you want a discussion of how amino acids transport through the intestinal wall.

Nutrient Utilization During Exercise. Report of the Ross Symposium. Ross Laboratories, Columbus, Ohio 43216. This book contains all you'd ever want to know about the most up-to-date information on the utilization of fat, protein, and carbohydrate during exercise.

Nutritive Value of American Foods in Common Units. Agriculture Handbook No. 456, U.S. Department of Agriculture. $8.50. I used this book as one of the basic sources for the Fat, Protein, Carbohydrate Content tables listed in the Appendix. You can obtain a copy by writing: Superintendent of Documents, U.S. Government Printing Office, Washington, D.C. 20402.

APPENDIX

Calorie/Protein/Fat/ Carbohydrate Content of Commonly Used Foods

FOOD	CALORIES	PROTEIN (g)	FAT (g)	CARBO-HYDRATE (g)
Almonds, 12–15 nuts	90	2.8	8.1	2.9
chopped, 1 tbs.	48	1.5	4.3	1.6
roasted, 1 oz.	176	5.2	16.2	5.5
whole, 1 cup	849	26.4	77	27.7
Almond paste, 1 oz.	144	3.1	9.1	14.5
Apple, raw 3-inch fruit				
(6½ oz.)	96	0.3	1.0	24
½ fruit (4 oz.)	61	0.2	0.6	15.3
canned, sliced sweetened,				
½ cup	68	0.2	0.5	17
dried, sulfured, 10 rings	155	0.6	0.2	42.4
micro-cooked, no skin,				
1 cup	96	0.5	0.7	24.5
Apple butter, 1 tbs.	33	0.1	0.1	8.2
Applesauce, 1 cup				
sweetened	194	0.4	0.4	51
1 cup unsweetened	100	0.5	0.5	26.4
Apricots, raw, 3 medium	55	1.1	0.2	13.7

FOOD	CALORIES	PROTEIN (g)	FAT (g)	CARBO-HYDRATE (g)
4 halves canned in syrup	75	0.5	0.1	19.3
3 halves, juice pack	40	0.5	tr	10.4
10 dried halves	91	1.8	0.2	23.3
frozen, sweetened, ½ cup	119	0.9	0.1	30.4
Alfalfa sprouts, 3½ oz.	41	5.1	0.6	5.5
Artichoke, 1 globe, 3 oz.	44	2.8	0.2	9.9
frozen hearts, ½ cup	32	2.3	0.4	6.6
Asparagus, 4 med. spears	12	1.3	0.1	2.2
pieces, ⅔ cup	20	2.2	0.2	3.6
canned, ½ cup	16	1.8	0.2	4.2
Avocado, Calif., 10 oz.	369	4.7	36.7	12.9
Florida, 16 oz.	389	4	33.4	26.7
Bacon, bits, Oscar Mayer, ¼ oz.	20	2.4	1	0.2
Canadian, 1 oz.	58	5.7	3.7	0.1
cured, fried crisp, 2 sl.	86	3.8	7.8	0.5
fresh raw fat, 1 oz.	177	2	18.6	0
Baking powder	3	tr	tr	0.7
Baking soda	–	–	–	–
Bamboo shoots, 1 cup	41	4	0.3	tr
Banana, 1 med., 8-inch	101	1.3	0.2	26.4
flakes, ½ cup	170	2	0.5	44.5
Barbecue sauce, 1 cup	228	3.8	17.3	20
Barley, 1 oz. dry, ½ cup cooked	98	2.9	tr	22.1
Beans, mature seeds, cooked				
black, 1 cup	225	15	1	41
Great Northern, 1 cup	210	14	1	38
lima, 1 cup	260	16	1	49
navy, 1 cup	225	15	1	40
pinto, 1 cup	265	15	1	49
canned in tomato sauce, 1 cup	232	11.4	1.8	42.7
pork & beans, 1 cup	250	11.4	3.9	42.7
beans & molasses, 1 cup	251	12.8	0.9	47.7
Beans, lima, immature seeds, 1 cup	189	12	0.9	33.7

FOOD	CALORIES	PROTEIN (g)	FAT (g)	CARBO-HYDRATE (g)
Beans, green snap, 1 cup	35	2.1	0.2	7.8
Italian, ⅔ cup	22	1.2	0.1	5.1
French w/ toasted almonds, ½ cup	52	2.5	1.6	8.4
Green bean & mushroom casserole, ½ cup	150	4	9	12
Bean sprouts (mung), 1 cup	37	4	0.2	6.9
Beef, chipped, 3 oz.	173	29.1	5.4	0
brisket, 3 oz.	411	17.3	37.4	0
chuck roast, 3 oz.	325	22	26	0
ground chuck, 3 oz.	327	26	23.9	0
club steak, 3 oz.	260	23.9	17.5	0
corned beef, 3½ oz.	372	22.9	30.4	0
cubed steak, 3½ oz.	261	28.6	15.4	0
flank steak, 5 oz.	331	47.1	14.4	0
meatballs, 1 oz.	70	3	5	0
meatloaf, 3½ oz.	160	17	7.6	4.6
porterhouse steak, 3½ oz.	242	25.4	14.7	0
rib roast, 3½ oz.	264	28.4	16.7	0
ribeye, 3½ oz.	440	19.9	39.4	0
bottom round, 3 oz.	220	25	13	0
top round, 4 oz.	254	43.1	5.9	0
ground round, 4 oz.	202	23.4	11.3	0
rump roast, 4 oz.	231	36	8.4	0
salisbury steak/gravy, 8 oz.	364	17.3	12.3	12.1
short ribs, 2½ oz.	290	17.6	23.9	0
sirloin, 4 oz.	355	19.1	30.2	0
T-bone, 3½ oz.	235	24	14.7	0
tenderloin, 2⅓ oz.	148	17.2	8.3	0
Beets, 2 medium raw	43	1.6	0.1	9.9
diced, cooked, 1 cup	84	2.2	0.2	19.4
pickled, 1 cup sliced	180	2	0	45
greens, ½ cup cooked	18	1.7	0.2	3.3
Beverages, alcoholic				
ale, 8 oz.	98	1.1	0	0
beer, regular, 8 oz.	151	1.1	0	13.7
beer, light, 12 oz.	100	0.4	0	6

FOOD	CALORIES	PROTEIN (g)	FAT (g)	CARBO-HYDRATE (g)
cordials & liqueurs, 54 proof, 1 oz.	97	0	0	11.5
daiquiri, 3½ oz.	122	0.1	0	5.2
eggnog, 4 oz.	335	3.9	15.8	18
gin, rum, vodka, 80 proof, 1 oz.	65	0	0	tr
gin rickey, 4 oz.	150	tr	0	1.3
manhattan, 3⅓ oz.	164	tr	0	7.9
martini, 3½ oz.	140	0.1	0	0.3
planter's punch, 3½ oz.	175	0.1	0	7.9
tom collins, 10 oz.	180	0.3	0	9
whiskey sour, 2½ oz.	138	0.2	0	7.7
champagne, 4 oz.	84	0.2	0	0.3
dessert wine, sweet, 3½ oz.	153	0.1	0	11.4
port, 3½ oz.	158	0.2	0	14
sauterne, 3½ oz.	84	0.2	0	4
sherry, 2 oz.	84	0.2	0	4.8
red table wine, 3½ oz.	75	tr	0	3
white table wine, 3½ oz.	80	tr	0	3
vermouth, dry, 3½ oz.	105	0	0	1
Beverages, non-alcoholic				
bitter lemon, 12 oz.	192	0	0	47.3
cola, 12 oz.	183	0	0	45.7
cream soda, 12 oz.	156	0	0	40.5
ginger ale, 12 oz.	113	0	0	29
grape soda, 12 oz.	179	0	0	45.8
lemon-lime, 12 oz.	144	0	0	39.6
orange soda, 12 oz.	179	0	0	45.8
quinine water, 4 oz.	37	0	0	9.6
rootbeer, 12 oz.	162	0	0	42.2
tonic water, 4 oz.	42	0	0	10.4
Biscuits, homemade, 2-inch refrigerated dough, 1	91	2	3.1	13.6
Blackberries, 1 cup fresh	84	1.7	1.3	18.6
canned in syrup, ½ cup	118	1.7	0.2	29.6
Blackeyed peas, 1 cup	184	13.1	1.2	31.6
Blueberries, 1 cup fresh	90	1	0.7	22.2
canned in syrup, ½ cup	112	0.8	0.4	28.2

FOOD	CALORIES	PROTEIN (g)	FAT (g)	CARBO- HYDRATE (g)
Bouillon cube	5	0.8	0.1	0.2
Boysenberries, frozen,				
plain, 1 cup	66	1.5	0.4	16.1
canned in syrup, ½ cup	113	1.3	0.2	28.6
Brazil nuts, 1 cup	916	20	93.7	15.3
4 medium	97	2.2	9.9	1.7
Breads, bagel, 2 oz. plain	150	6	1	30
bagel, 2 oz. raisin	200	8	1	40
cracked wheat, 1 slice	66	2.2	0.6	13.0
French bread, 1 slice	51	1.6	0.5	9.7
fruit/nut quick bread,				
1 slice	118	1.8	2.4	22.3
Italian, 1 slice	55	1.8	0.2	11.3
matzo, 1 piece	117	3	0.3	25.4
mixed grain, 1 slice	64	2.5	0.9	11.7
raisin, 1 slice	66	1.7	0.7	13.4
pumpernickel, 1 slice	79	2.9	0.4	17
sourdough, 1 slice	68	2.5	0.5	13.4
spoon bread, 3½ oz.	187	6.4	10.9	16.2
wheat, 1 slice	61	2.3	1	11.3
wheatberry, 1 slice	70	2.5	1.1	12.3
white, 1 slice	68	2.2	0.6	10.1
white, homemade,				
1 slice	72	1.9	1.7	12
Bread crumbs, 1 cup	345	11.1	4	64.6
Bread sticks, reg. 1 stick	23	0.7	0.3	4.5
garlic, 1 stick	24	0.7	0.3	3.4
Broccoli, raw, 1 stalk	32	3.6	0.3	5.9
cooked, ⅔ cup	26	3.1	0.3	4.5
au gratin, 5 oz.	170	7	12	9
Brussels sprouts (6–8 med.)	36	4.2	0.4	6.4
cooked, 1 cup	56	6.5	0.6	9.9
au gratin, 5½ oz.	180	6	11	16
Buckwheat flour, 1 cup				
sifted	340	6.3	1.2	77.9
Bulgur, 1 cup dry	602	19	2.6	128.7
Butter, 1 tbs.	102	0.1	11.5	0.1
1 stick, ½ cup	812	0.7	91.9	0.5
1 cup	1625	1.4	183.9	0.9

FOOD	CALORIES	PROTEIN (g)	FAT (g)	CARBO-HYDRATE (g)
whipped type, 1 stick	541	0.5	61.2	0.3
whipped type, 1 cup	1081	0.9	122.3	0.6
Butter beans, ½ cup	138	7.5	0.6	26.3
Cabbage, Chinese raw, 2¼ cup	14	1.2	0.1	3
Chinese cooked, ½ cup	8	1.2	0	1.3
green raw, 1 cup	22	1.2	0.2	4.9
green cooked, ⅗ cup	20	1.1	0.2	4.3
red raw, 1 cup shredded	31	2	0.2	6.9
savory raw, 1 cup shredded	12	1.2	0.1	2.3
Cakes, angelfood, 1/12 tube	161	4.3	0.1	36.1
applesauce spice, 1/12	250	3	11	34
Sara Lee apple walnut, ⅛	212	2.3	10.2	27.7
banana, 1/12	260	3	11	36
Sara Lee black forest, ⅛	194	1.8	9.3	27.9
Boston cream, 4 oz.	332	5.5	10.3	54.9
butter pecan, 1/12	250	3	11	35
butter recipe mix, 1/12	230	3	8	36
caramel, mix, 1/12	173	2	7.8	24.2
carrot, mix, 1/12	250	3	11	35
Sara Lee carrot, ⅛	238	2.5	12.1	29.4
cheesecake, mix, ⅛	300	6	14.3	37.8
chocolate, mix, 1/12	250	3	11	35
devil's food, homemade, 1/12	227	3.4	11.3	30.4
devil's food w/frosting, 1/12	233	2.6	10.1	34.2
dark fruitcake, 1½ oz.	152	1.9	6.1	23.9
light fruitcake, 1½ oz.	156	2.4	6.6	23
German chocolate, 1/12	260	3	11	36
gingerbread, homemade, 3 × 3-inch	371	4.4	12.5	60.8
mix, 1/9 cake	210	2	6	36
lemon, mix, 1/12	260	3	11	36
lemon chiffon, mix, 1/12	190	4	4	35
marble, mix, 1/12	270	3	11	40
pineapple upside-down, 1/9	236	2.5	9.1	37.4

FOOD	CALORIES	PROTEIN (g)	FAT (g)	CARBO-HYDRATE (g)
plum pudding, 2-inch wedge	270	4	1	61
pound, homemade, 1 oz.	142	1.7	8.8	14.1
pound, mix, 1 oz.	125	1.6	6.9	14.2
shortcake, 1 oz.	86	1	2	12
Duncan Hines snack cake, ⅑	187	2.3	5.3	31.7
sponge, 2½ oz.	188	4.8	3.1	35.7
white, sheet, 3 × 3-inch	315	4	12	48
yellow, 2½ oz.	283	4.3	12.4	38.9
Hostess chocolate cup-cakes, 2	314	2.9	8.8	58.8
Hostess orange cup-cakes, 2	294	2.5	8.4	52.9
Hostess Ho Hos, 2	235	2.2	11.8	32.5
Hostess Snoballs, 2	269	2.5	7.6	49.6
Hostess Twinkies, 2	286	2.5	8.4	51.2
Candy, Butterscotch, 6 pieces	116	0	2.5	24.3
butterscotch chips, 1 oz.	150	1	7	19
caramels, 1 oz.	113	1	2.9	21.7
chocolate, bittersweet, 1 oz.	135	2.2	11.3	13.3
chocolate, semisweet, 1 cup	862	7	60	97
chocolate, semisweet, 1 oz.	144	1.2	10	16
chocolate, sweet, 1 oz.	150	1.2	10	16.4
milk chocolate, 1 oz.	151	2.6	10	14.5
milk chocolate w/peanuts, 1 oz.	154	4	10.8	12.6
fudge, 1 oz.	122	1.1	4.5	20.7
fudge w/nuts, 1 oz.	128	1.4	5.9	19.1
candy corn, 1 cup	728	0.2	4	179.2
fondant mints, 1½ rounds	32	tr	0.2	7.9
vanilla fudge, 1 oz.	113	.9	3.1	21.2
vanilla fudge w/nuts, 1 oz.	120	1.2	4.6	19.5
gum drops, 1 oz.	98	tr	0.2	24.8

FOOD	CALORIES	PROTEIN (g)	FAT (g)	CARBO-HYDRATE (g)
jellybeans, 1 cup	807	tr	1.1	204.8
jellybeans (10 pieces)	104	tr	0.1	26.4
marshmallow, large	23	.1	tr	5.8
marshmallow, miniature, 1 cup	147	.9	tr	37
peanut brittle, 1 oz.	119	1.6	2.9	23
malted milk balls, 14	135	2.3	7	17.8
English toffee, 1 oz.	193	.9	16.7	9.7
chocolate-covered raisins, 1 oz.	115	1	3.7	19.5
chocolate-covered peanuts, 1 oz.	153	4.6	9	13.3
Life Savers, 5 pieces	39	0	0.1	9.7
Reese's pieces, 1.7 oz.	240	7.1	10	30
sugar-coated almonds, 7	128	2.2	5.2	19.7
Carrot, whole raw 7-inch	30	0.8	0.1	7
raw, 1 cup grated	46	1.2	0.2	10.7
cooked, 1 cup sliced	48	1.4	0.3	11
canned, 1 cup	69	1.5	0.5	16
dehydrated, 1 oz.	97	1.9	0.4	23
Cantaloupe, ½ 5-inch melon	82	1.9	0.3	20.4
frozen, 3.5 cup	31	0.8	tr	7.7
Cashews, roasted, 6–8 nuts	84	2.6	6.9	4.4
1 cup, dry-roasted	785	21	63	45
Cauliflower, 1 cup raw	23	2.3	0.2	4.4
cooked, ⅞ cup	22	2.3	0.2	4.1
au gratin, 5 oz.	155	6	1	11
Caviar, granular, 1 tbs.	43	4.3	2.4	0.5
granular, 1 oz.	74	7.6	4.3	0.9
pressed, 1 tbs.	54	5.8	2.8	0.8
pressed, 1 oz.	90	9.8	4.7	1.4
Celery, green raw, large 8-inch stalk	7	0.4	tr	1.6
small inner 5-inch	9	0.5	0.1	2
1 cup chopped	20	1.1	0.1	4.7
Cereals, corn grits, 1 cup cooked	145	3	tr	31
Cream of Wheat, 1 cup	140	4	tr	29
Malt-O-Meal, 1 cup	120	4	tr	26

FOOD	CALORIES	PROTEIN (g)	FAT (g)	CARBO-HYDRATE (g)
oatmeal, 1 cup	145	6	2	25
instant oatmeal w/apple-cinn., 1 pkg. prepared	135	3.9	1.6	26.3
Ralston, ¾ cup cooked	100	4.2	0.6	21.2
Wheatena, ¾ cup cooked	101	3.7	0.8	21.5
All-Bran, 1 oz.	70	4	1	21
Bran Buds, 1 oz.	73	3.9	0.7	21.6
Cherrios, 1 oz.	110	4	2	20
Bran Chex, 1 oz.	91	2.9	0.8	22.6
Bran Flakes, 1 oz.	93	3.6	0.5	22.2
Buc Wheats, 1 oz.	108	2	1	22.7
Cap'n Crunch, 1 oz.	119	1.5	2.6	22.9
Cocoa Krispies, 1 oz.	110	1.5	0.4	25.2
Corn Bran, 1 oz.	98	1.9	1	23.9
Corn Chex, 1 oz.	111	2	0.1	24.9
Corn Flakes, 1 oz.	110	2	tr	24
Fruit Loops, 1 oz.	110	2	1	25
granola, homemade, 1 oz.	138	3.5	7.7	15.6
GrapeNuts, 1 oz.	100	3	tr	23
Product 19, 1 oz.	108	2.8	0.2	23.5
Raisin Bran, 1 oz.	90	3	1	21
Puffed Rice, 1 oz.	57	0.9	0.1	12.8
Rice Krispies, 1 oz.	110	2	tr	25
Shredded Wheat, 1 oz.	100	3	1	23
Special K, 1 oz.	111	5.6	0.1	21.3
Total, 1 oz.	100	3	1	22
Nutri-Grain wheat & raisin, 1 oz.	140	3	0	33
Wheat Germ, toasted, 1 oz.	108	8.3	3	14.1
Wheaties, 1 oz.	100	3	tr	23
puffed wheat, 1 oz.	104	4.2	0.4	22.6
Quaker, 100% natural, 1 oz.	133	3.3	6.1	17.8
Quaker, 100% natural, w/ raisins & dates, 1 oz.	128	2.9	5.2	18.7
Chard, Swiss, leaves, cooked, 1 cup	32	3.2	0.4	5.8

FOOD	CALORIES	PROTEIN (g)	FAT (g)	CARBO-HYDRATE (g)
leaves & stalks, 1 cup	26	2.6	0.3	4.8
Charlotte russe, 1 serving, 4 oz.	326	6.7	16.6	38.2
Cheese, blue, 1 oz.	104	6.1	8.6	0.6
brie, 1 oz.	95	5.9	7.9	0.1
brick, 1 oz.	105	6.3	8.6	0.5
camembert, 1 oz.	85	5	7	0.5
cheddar, 1 oz.	113	7.1	9.1	0.6
cheddar, grated, 1 cup	455	28.1	37.5	1.5
colby, 1 oz.	112	6.7	9.1	0.7
cottage, reg. 4.2%, 1 cup	239	30.9	9.5	6.5
cottage, low-fat, 2%, 1 cup	205	31	4	8
cottage, 1%, 1 cup	162	28	2.3	6.2
cottage, dry curd, 1 cup	112	25	0.6	2.6
cream, 1 oz. (2 tbs.)	104	2.2	10.6	0.6
edam, 1 oz.	101	7.1	7.9	0.4
gouda, 1 oz.	101	7.1	7.8	0.6
limburger, 1 oz.	98	6	7.9	0.6
Monterey Jack, 1 oz.	106	6.9	8.6	0.2
mozzarella, 1 oz.	80	5.5	6.1	0.6
mozzarella, low-moisture, 1 oz.	90	6.1	7	0.7
mozzarella, part-skim, 1 oz.	72	6.9	4.5	0.8
muenster, 1 oz.	104	6.6	8.5	0.3
neufchâtel, 1 oz.	74	2.8	6.6	0.8
Parmesan, 1 tbs.	21	1.9	1.4	0.2
provolone, 1 oz.	100	7.3	7.6	0.6
ricotta, part-skim, ½ cup	171	14.1	9.8	6.4
ricotta, whole milk, ½ cup	216	14	16.1	3.8
Romano, 1 oz.	110	9	7.6	1
Swiss, 1 oz.	107	8.1	7.8	1
American, 1 oz.	106	6.3	8.9	0.5
Velveeta, 1 oz.	80	5	6	2
pimiento cheese, 1 oz.	106	6.3	8.8	0.5
Cheese sauce, 2 tbs.	66	3	4.9	2.4
¼ cup	132	6	9.8	4.8

FOOD	CALORIES	PROTEIN (g)	FAT (g)	CARBO-HYDRATE (g)
Cherries, fresh sweet, 10	47	0.9	0.2	11.7
sour canned in water, ½ cup	43	0.9	0.1	10.9
sour in syrup, ½ cup	116	0.9	0.1	29.8
maraschino, 2 medium	19	tr	tr	4.7
Chicken, ½ breast w/skin, fried	218	31.2	8.7	1.6
½ breast w/skin, roasted	193	29.2	7.6	0
½ breast w/skin, stewed	202	30.1	8.2	0
½ breast w/o skin, fried	161	28.8	4.1	0.4
½ breast w/o skin, roasted	142	26.7	3.1	0
½ breast w/o skin, stewed	144	27.5	2.9	0
drumstick w/skin, fried	120	13.2	6.7	0.8
drumstick w/skin, roasted	112	14.1	5.8	0
drumstick w/o skin, roasted	76	12.5	2.5	0
thigh w/ skin, roasted	153	15.5	9.6	0
thigh w/o skin, roasted	109	13.5	5.7	0
capon, w/skin, roasted, 3½ oz.	229	29	11.7	0
canned, 2½ oz., light meat	117	15.5	5.6	0
canned, 2½ oz., dark meat	120	15	7	0
Chicken roll, light meat, 3½ oz.	159	19.5	7.4	2.5
Chicken à la king, 1 cup	468	27.4	34.3	12.3
Chicken parmigiana, 7 oz.	308	21.6	14.8	22.1
Chicken pie, Swanson, 8 oz.	450	14	25	41
homemade, 4 oz.	273	11.7	15.7	21.1
Chicken chow mein, 1 cup	224	27.3	8.8	8.8
Chives, 1 tsp.	tr	tr	tr	0.1
Chocolate syrup, 1 oz.	92	0.9	0.8	23.5
Clams, soft, raw, 4	82	14	1.9	1.3
hard, round, 5	80	11.1	0.9	5.9
canned, solids only, ½ cup	98	15.8	2.5	1.9

FOOD	CALORIES	PROTEIN (g)	FAT (g)	CARBO-HYDRATE (g)
canned, liquor only, ½ cup	19	2.3	0.1	2.1
Collards, 1 cup cooked	63	6.8	1.3	9.1
raw, 1 pound	255	27.2	4.5	42.5
Cookies, animal, 15	120	1.9	2.9	22
arrowroot, 2	47	0.6	1.7	7.3
brownie w/nuts, 3 × 1-inch frozen w/icing	97	1.3	6.3	10.2
1½ × 1 × ¾-inch	103	1.2	5	14.9
Pepperidge Farm Capri, 1	82	0.8	4.6	9.7
chocolate chip, homemade, 2⅓-inch	52	0.5	0.8	10.5
Pepperidge Farm Chocolate chip, 2	321	3.2	14.7	44.2
chocolate sandwich, 1	49	0.5	2.1	7.1
chocolate snaps, 4	53	0.7	1.8	8.8
coconut bar	109	1.4	5.4	14.1
fig bar	53	0.5	1	10.6
gingersnap, 2-inch	29	0.3	0.6	5.5
graham cracker, 2 squares	55	1.1	1.3	10.4
chocolate-covered graham, 1 cookie	62	0.7	3.1	8.8
Pepperidge Farm granola, 2 large	318	3.8	15.4	41
lemon cookies, 2	57	0.5	2.2	8.7
Pepperidge Farm lemon nut, 2 large	336	3.8	17.9	40.3
macaroon, 1	67	0.7	3.2	9.3
molasses, 1	71	0.8	2.9	10.2
oatmeal, homemade, 1	80	1.1	3.2	12.2
Little Debbie oatmeal creams, 2	332	3.7	12.6	51.1
oatmeal w/raisins, 1	59	0.8	2	9.5
peanut cookie, 1	57	0.3	2.3	8
peanut butter, 3-inch	50	0.8	2.6	5.9
shortbread, 1⅝-inch	37	0.5	1.7	4.8
sugar, 2¼-inch	35	0.4	1.3	5.4
sugar wafer, 3½ × 1-inch	46	0.4	1.8	6.9
vanilla wafer	18	0.2	0.6	2.9

FOOD	CALORIES	PROTEIN (g)	FAT (g)	CARBO-HYDRATE (g)
vienna finger sandwich	72	0.7	3	10.7
Corn, white, 1 cup	100	3	0.5	24.3
cream style, 1 cup	210	5.4	1.5	51.2
on the cob, 4-inch ear	100	3.3	1	21
yellow canned, 1 cup	169	4.9	1.9	40.3
Corn flour, 1 cup	431	9.1	3	89.9
Cornbread, 1 piece, 2½ × 2½ × 1½	161	5.8	5.6	22.7
Cornmeal, 1 cup	433	11.2	4.8	89.9
Corn salad, raw, 3½ oz.	21	2	0.4	3.9
Cornstarch, 1 tbs.	29	tr	tr	7
Crackers, butter	15	0.2	0.5	2.2
cheese, 1-inch sq., 10	52	1.2	2.3	6.5
saltine, 2	24	0.5	0.7	4
saltine crumbs, 1 cup	409	9.5	18.1	51.3
cheese/peanut butter sandwich, packet of 4	139	4.3	6.8	15.9
oyster, 10	33	0.7	1	5.3
Cranberries, raw, 1 cup	44	0.4	0.7	10.3
canned sauce, 1 cup	404	0.3	0.7	103.9
juice, 1 cup	164	0.3	0.3	41.7
Cream puff, 3½-inch, w/custard	303	8.5	18.1	26.7
Cream, half & half, 1 tbs.	20	0.5	1.8	0.7
1 cup	324	7.7	28.3	11.1
light, 1 cup	506	7.2	49.4	10.3
heavy or whipping, 1 tbs.	53	0.3	5.6	0.5
1 cup (2 cups whipped)	835	5.2	89.5	7.4
sour, 1 tbs.	25	tr	3	1.6
Cress, garden, raw, 5–8 sprigs	31	2.6	0.8	5.1
Crowder peas, ⅔ cup	126	7.7	0.9	22.7
Cucumber, raw, 6-inch	25	1.5	0.2	5.8
sliced, 1 cup	16	0.9	0.1	3.6
Custard, baked, 1 cup	305	14.3	14.6	29.4
Dandelion greens, 1 cup cooked	204	12.2	3.2	41.7
Dates, 10 whole	219	1.8	0.4	58.3

FOOD	CALORIES	PROTEIN (g)	FAT (g)	CARBO-HYDRATE (g)
chopped, 1 cup	488	3.9	0.9	129.8
Doughnuts, cake, 2 oz.	227	2.7	10.8	29.8
yeast, 1½ oz.	176	2.7	11.3	16
Eggs, raw, whole, x-large	94	7.4	6.6	0.5
large	82	6.5	5.8	0.5
medium	72	5.7	5.1	0.4
1 cup	396	31.3	27.9	2.2
white of large egg	17	3.6	tr	0.3
1 cup whites	124	26.5	0.1	1.9
yolk of large egg	59	2.7	5.2	0.1
1 cup yolks	846	38.9	74.4	1.5
duck, whole raw	134	9.4	10.2	0.5
goose, whole raw	266	20	19.1	1.9
Eggplant, 1 cup diced	38	2	0.4	8.2
Endive, 1 cup	10	0.9	0.1	2.1
Fig, large	52	0.8	0.2	13.2
medium	40	0.6	0.2	10.2
small	32	0.5	0.1	8.1
canned in syrup, 1 cup	218	1.3	0.5	56.5
Filberts (hazelnuts) 1 cup	856	17	84.2	22.5
10 whole	87	1.7	8.6	2.3
Fish, abalone, 3½ oz.	98	18.7	0.5	3.4
bass, freshwater, 3½ oz.	104	18.9	2.6	0
bass, saltwater, 3½ oz.	100	18.9	2.7	0
bluefish, 3½ oz.	117	20.5	3.3	0
bonito, 3½ oz.	257	19.8	19.1	0
catfish, 3½ oz.	103	17.6	3.1	0
cod, 3½ oz.	78	17.6	0.3	0
crab, steamed, 3½ oz.	93	17.3	1.9	0.5
crappie, 3½ oz.	79	16.8	0.8	0
flounder/sole, 3½ oz.	68	14.9	0.5	0
haddock, 3½ oz.	79	18.2	0.1	0
halibut, 3½ oz.	100	20.9	1.2	0
lake trout, 3½ oz.	241	14.3	19.9	0
rainbow trout, 3½ oz.	195	21.5	11.4	0
lobster, 3½ oz.	91	16.9	1.9	0.5
mackerel, 3½ oz.	191	19	12.2	0
oysters, 6 raw	66	8.4	1.8	3.4
canned, 3½ oz.	76	8.5	2.2	4.9

FOOD	CALORIES	PROTEIN (g)	FAT (g)	CARBO-HYDRATE (g)
fried, 3½ oz.	239	8.6	13.9	18.6
scalloped, 6 medium	336	15.9	18	31.6
shrimp, 3½ oz.	91	18.8	0.8	1.5
fried, 3½ oz.	225	20.3	10.8	10
salmon, raw, 3½ oz.	217	22.5	13.4	0
smoked, 3½ oz.	176	21.6	9.3	0
swordfish, 3½ oz.	118	19.2	4	0
tuna, water-packed, 6½ oz.	237	51.5	3.5	0.1
packed w/oil, 6½ oz.	386	46.9	22.1	0.2
Fruit cocktail, water-packed, 1 cup	91	1	0.2	23.8
syrup-packed, 1 cup	194	1	0.3	50.2
Goose, w/skin, roasted, 3½ oz.	305	25.2	21.9	0
w/o skin, roasted, 3½ oz.	238	29	12.7	0
Gooseberries, 1 cup	59	1.2	0.3	14.6
Grapefruit, ½ of 3½-inch fruit	40	0.5	0.1	10.3
1 cup sections	82	1	0.2	21.2
juice, 1 cup	96	1.2	0.2	22.6
Grapes, seedless, 10	34	0.3	0.2	8.7
w/seeds, 10	38	0.3	0.2	9.9
juice, frozen reconst., 1 cup	133	0.5	tr	33.3
Honey, 1 tbs.	64	0.1	0	17.3
Honeydew melon, ¹⁄₁₀ of 7-inch melon	49	1.2	0.4	11.5
Horseradish, 1 tsp.	2	0.1	tr	0.5
Ice cream, reg. 10% fat, 1 cup	257	6	14.1	27.7
soft serve, 1 cup	334	7.8	18.3	36
rich, 16% fat, 1 cup	329	3.8	23.8	26.6
Ice milk, 5.1% fat, 1 cup	199	6.3	6.7	29.3
soft serve, 1 cup	266	8.4	8.9	39.2
Ice, lime, 1 cup	247	0.8	tr	62.9
Jam, 1 tbs.	54	0.1	tr	14
Jelly, 1 tbs.	49	tr	tr	12.7
Kale, 1 cup cooked	43	5	0.8	6.7

FOOD	CALORIES	PROTEIN (g)	FAT (g)	CARBO-HYDRATE (g)
Kohlrabi, 1 cup diced	41	2.8	0.1	9.2
Kumquat, 1 medium	12	0.2	tr	3.2
Lamb, arm chop, 3½ oz.	339	22.4	27	0
blade chop, 3½ oz.	340	24.6	26.1	0
leg, roasted, 3½ oz.	242	20.6	14.5	0
loin chop, 1.6 oz.	103	12.5	5.5	0
rib chop, 1½ oz.	119	10.5	8.3	0
Lard, 1 cup	1849	0	205	0
Lemon, pulp of large	29	1.2	0.2	8.7
juice, 1 tbs.	4	0.1	tr	1.2
Lemonade, 1 cup	107	0.1	tr	28.3
Lentils, 1 cup cooked	212	15.6	tr	28.3
Lettuce, butterhead,				
lg. leaf	2	0.2	tr	0.4
crisphead, lg. leaf	3	0.2	tr	0.6
cos/romaine, 1 cup	10	0.7	0.2	1.9
Lime, pulp of 2-inch fruit	19	0.5	0.1	6.4
juice, 1 tbs.	4	tr	tr	1.4
Limeade, 1 cup	102	0.1	tr	27
Liver, beef, 3 oz. fried	195	22.4	9	4.5
calf, 3 oz. fried	222	25.1	11.2	3.4
beef raw, 3½ oz.	140	19.9	3.8	5.3
chicken, 1 liver raw	41	6.6	1.1	0.8
turkey, 1 liver from 20-lb.				
bird	212	34	5.9	3.8
Loganberries, 1 cup	89	1.4	0.9	21.5
Loquats, 10	59	0.5	0.2	15.3
Macaroni, 2 oz. dry	209	7.1	0.6	42.5
Macaroni & cheese, 1 cup	430	16.8	22.2	40.2
Mango, 10-oz. fruit	152	1.6	0.9	38.8
Malt, dry, 1 oz.	104	0.3	0.5	21.9
Malt extract, 1 oz.	104	1.7	tr	25.3
Margarine, regular, 1 tbs.	102	0.1	11.5	0.1
1 cup	1634	1.4	183.9	0.9
whipped type, 1 tbs.	68	0.1	7.6	tr
1 cup	1087	0.9	122.3	0.6
Marmalade, 1 tbs.	51	0.1	tr	14
Mayonnaise, regular, 1 tbs.	101	0.2	11.2	0.3

FOOD	CALORIES	PROTEIN (g)	FAT (g)	CARBO-HYDRATE (g)
1 cup	1580	2.4	175.8	4.8
light, 1 tbs.	45	0	5	1
Milk, whole, 3.5%, 1 cup	159	8.5	8.5	12
low-fat, 2%, 1 cup	145	10.3	4.9	14.8
low-fat, 1%, 1 cup	102	8	2.6	11.7
skim, non-fat, 1 cup	88	8.8	0.2	12.5
canned, evap., 1 cup	345	17.6	19.9	24.4
evap. skim, 1 cup	200	19.2	0.8	28.8
sweetened cond., 1 cup	982	24.8	26.6	166.2
goat, 1 cup	163	7.8	9.8	11.2
human, 1 cup	168	2.4	11.2	16.8
sheep, 1 cup	264	14.7	17.2	13.1
soybean, 1 cup	87	8.9	4	5.8
malted powder, 1 oz.	116	4.2	2.4	20.1
chocolate whole, 1 cup	213	8.5	8.5	27.5
Molasses, 1 tbs.	50	0	0	13
Muffins, plain 3-inch	118	3.1	4	16.9
blueberry, 2⅜-inch	112	2.9	3.7	16.8
bran, 2⅝-inch	104	3.1	3.9	17.2
corn, 2⅜-inch	126	2.8	4	19.2
whole wheat, 2½-inch	103	4	1.1	20.9
English, 1	135	4.5	1.1	26.2
English w/raisins	146	4.5	2.2	27.4
English sourdough	129	4.5	1.1	25.2
Mushrooms, raw, 1 cup	20	1.9	0.2	3.1
canned, ⅓ cup	17	1.1	0.2	2.3
sautéed, 4 medium	78	1.7	7.4	2.8
Mustard greens, 1 cup cooked	32	3.1	0.6	5.6
Mustard, brown, 1 tsp.	5	0.3	0.3	0.3
yellow, 1 tsp.	4	0.2	0.2	0.3
Mustard spinach, 1 cup cooked	29	3.1	0.4	5
New Zealand spinach, 1 cup cooked	23	3.1	0.4	3.8
Nectarine, 2½-inch fruit	88	0.8	tr	23.6
Noodles, egg, 2 oz. dry	220	7.2	2.6	40.7
Noodles, chow mein, ½ cup	153	2.7	8.8	15.8

FOOD	CALORIES	PROTEIN (g)	FAT (g)	CARBO-HYDRATE (g)
rice, dry, 1 oz.	130	2	0.6	22.7
romanoff from mix, ¼ pkg.	230	7	12	23
Oil, corn, safflower, soy-bean, cottonseed, 1 cup	1927	0	218	0
1 tbs.	120	0	13.6	0
veg. oil spray, 2 sec.	8	0	0.8	0
Okra, 1 cup raw	36	2.4	0.3	7.8
1 cup boiled	46	3.2	0.5	9.6
Okra gumbo, 1 cup	225	2.2	17.5	14
Olives, green whole, 10 sm.	33	0.4	3.6	0.4
10 large	45	0.5	24	7
10 giant	76	0.9	40	11
ripe whole, 10 extra-lg.	61	0.5	6.5	1.2
10 mammoth	72	0.6	7.7	1.5
10 giant	89	0.8	9.5	1.8
Onions, mature, 1 cup chopped	65	2.6	0.2	14.8
1 cup grated	89	3.5	0.2	20.4
1 tbs. chopped	4	0.2	tr	0.9
1 cup cooked	61	2.5	0.2	13.7
Onion, green, 1 cup chopped	36	1.5	0.2	8.2
1 tbs. chopped	2	0.1	tr	0.5
Orange, navel, large, 9 oz.	87	2.2	0.2	21.8
medium, 7.3 oz.	71	1.8	0.1	17.8
small, 4.6 oz.	45	1.2	0.1	11.3
1 cup sections	77	2	0.2	19.1
Florida, large, 9.1 oz.	89	1.3	0.3	22.6
medium, 7.2 oz.	71	1.1	0.3	18.1
small, 5.8 oz.	57	0.8	0.2	14.5
sections, 1 cup	78	1.2	0.3	19.8
Orange juice, fresh, 1 cup	112	1.7	0.5	25.8
canned unsweetened, 1 cup	120	2	0.5	27.9
frozen, reconst., unsweet-ened, 1 cup	122	1.7	0.2	28.9
dried crystals, 1 oz.	108	1.4	0.5	25.2
Orange peel, 1 tbs.	0	0.1	tr	1.5

FOOD	CALORIES	PROTEIN (g)	FAT (g)	CARBO-HYDRATE (g)
Pancakes, egg and milk, 4-inch made w/2½ tbs. batter	61	1.9	2	8.7
buckwheat, same as above	54	1.8	2.5	6.4
blueberry, 4-inch	68	2.1	0.5	13.8
cornmeal, 4-inch	68	2.3	1.3	11.4
Papaya, whole 16 oz.	119	1.8	0.3	30.4
cubed, 1 cup	55	0.8	0.1	14
mashed, 1 cup	90	1.4	0.2	23
Parsley, 1 cup chopped	26	2.2	0.4	5.1
1 tbs. chopped	1	0.1	tr	0.3
10 sprigs	4	0.4	0.1	0.9
Parsnip, large cooked	106	2.4	0.8	23.8
small boiled (6-inch)	23	0.5	0.2	5.2
diced, 1 cup	102	2.3	0.6	23.1
mashed, 1 cup	139	3.2	1.1	31.3
Pawpaw, common raw, 2-inch	83	5.1	0.9	16.4
Peach, 2¾-inch	58	0.9	0.2	14.8
2½-inch	38	0.5	0.1	8.5
1 cup sliced	65	1	0.2	16.5
1 cup canned in syrup	200	1	0.3	51.5
dried, 10 large halves	380	4.5	1	99
dried, 10 medium halves	341	4	0.9	88.8
Peach nectar, 1 cup	120	0.5	tr	30.9
Peanuts, 1 cup chopped	838	37.7	70	29.7
10 Virginia nut or 20 Spanish	53	2.3	4.5	1.7
Peanut butter, 1 tbs.	94	4	8.1	3
Pear, 2½-inch Bartlett	100	1.1	0.7	25.1
2½-inch Bosc	86	1	0.6	21.6
3-inch Anjou	122	1.4	0.8	30.6
1 cup sliced	101	1.2	0.7	25.2
1 cup canned in syrup	194	0.5	0.5	50
dried, 10 halves	469	5.4	3.2	117.8
Pear nectar, 1 cup	130	0.8	0.5	33
Peas, green raw, 1 cup	122	9.1	0.6	20.9
1 cup cooked	114	8.6	0.6	19.4

FOOD	CALORIES	PROTEIN (g)	FAT (g)	CARBO-HYDRATE (g)
1 cup canned	164	8.7	0.7	31.1
creamed, ½ cup	136	4.5	6.9	14.2
peas & carrots, ⅗ cup	45	2.2	0.3	8.4
snow peas, 6 oz.	90	5.8	0.3	20.4
Split peas, 1 cup cooked	230	16	0.6	41.6
Pecans, shelled, 10 large				
halves	62	0.8.	6.4	1.3
10 jumbo halves	96	1.3	10	2
10 mammoth	124	1.7	1.8	2.6
1 cup	742	9.9	76.9	15.8
1 tbs. chopped	52	0.7	5.3	1.1
Peppers, hot chili sauce,				
1 cup	49	1.7	0.2	12.3
sweet green, 1, 3¾-inch	36	2	0.3	7.9
1 cup chopped	33	1.8	0.3	7.2
1 cup cooked	24	1.4	0.3	5.1
stuffed w/beef, crumbs	315	24.1	10.2	31.1
Persimmon, raw, Japanese	129	1.2	0.7	33.1
Pickle, whole dill, 4-inch	15	0.9	0.3	3
1 cup slices	17	1.1	0.3	3.4
gherkin, large 3-inch	51	0.2	0.1	12.8
small, 2½-inch	22	0.1	0.1	5.5
midget, 2⅛-inch	9	tr	tr	2.2
chopped, 1 cup	234	1.1	0.6	58.4
chowchow, sour, 1 cup	70	3.4	3.1	9.8
sweet, 1 cup	284	3.7	2.2	66.2
relish, 1 cup	338	1.2	1.5	83.3
1 tbs.	21	0.1	0.1	5.1
Pie, ⅛ of 9-inch pie				
apple	302	2.6	13.1	45
banana custard	252	5.1	10.6	35
blackberry	287	3.1	13	40.6
blueberry	286	2.8	12.7	41.2
cherry	308	3.1	13.3	45.3
chocolate meringue	287	5.5	13.7	38.2
chocolate chiffon	266	5.5	12.4	35.4
chocolate cream	301	5.2	17.3	33.6
coconut custard	249	7	12.7	26.7
coconut cream	270	2	14	33

FOOD	CALORIES	PROTEIN (g)	FAT (g)	CARBO-HYDRATE (g)
lemon chiffon	254	5.7	10.2	35.5
lemon meringue	268	3.9	10.7	39.6
lemon cream	245	2	12	32
mincemeat	320	3	13.6	48.3
peach	301	3	12.6	45.1
pecan	431	5.3	23.6	52.8
pineapple	299	2.6	12.6	45
pumpkin	241	4.6	12.8	27.9
raisin	319	3.1	12.6	50.7
rhubarb	299	3	12.6	45.1
strawberry w/whipped cream	378	2.9	16.8	56.2
sweet potato	342	7.2	18.2	37.8
Piecrust, 1 shell	900	11	60	78.8
Pigs' feet, pickled 2 oz.	113	9.5	8.4	0
Pimientos, 4-oz. jar.	31	1	0.6	6.6
Pineapple, 1 cup raw	81	0.6	0.3	21.2
canned, syrup, 1 cup	189	0.8	0.3	49.2
canned, juice pack, 1 cup	150	1	0.2	39.2
juice, unsweetened, 1 cup	138	1	0.3	33.8
juice, with grapefruit, 1 cup	135	0.5	0.1	34
juice w/orange, 1 cup	135	0.5	0.3	33.8
Pinenuts, 1 oz.	156	8.8	13.4	3.3
Pistachios, 30 nuts	88	2.9	8	2.8
Pizza, homemade, 14-inch cheese	153	7.8	5.4	18.4
sausage	157	5.2	6.2	19.8
pepperoni, ¼ Celeste	356	16.3	27	18.2
sausage & mushroom, ¼ Celeste	379	16.9	19.3	34.3
Plum, raw, damson, 10	66	0.5	tr	17.8
1 cup pitted halves	112	0.9	tr	30.3
Japanese, 2½-inch	32	0.3	0.1	8.1
1 cup pitted halves	89	0.9	0.4	22.8
prune type, 1½-inch	21	0.2	0.1	5.6
1 cup halves	124	1.3	0.8	32.5
canned w/syrup, 1 cup	215	1	0.3	57.8
Pomegranate, raw, 3⅜-inch	97	0.8	0.5	25.3

FOOD	CALORIES	PROTEIN (g)	FAT (g)	CARBO-HYDRATE (g)
Popcorn, 1 cup unpopped	742	24.4	9.6	147.8
popped, plain, 1 cup	28	0.8	0.3	4.6
oil & salt added, 1 cup	41	0.9	2	5.3
sugar-coated, 1 cup	134	2.1	1.2	29.9
Popover, 2¾-inch	90	3.5	3.7	10.3
Pork, blade lean slice, 2.1 oz.	134	18.8	5.9	0
boston butt, lean, 2.9 oz.	162	23.6	7	0
ham, lean, 2.6 oz.	167	29	4.8	0
cured ham, lean, 2.3 oz.	102	17.7	2.9	0.2
canned ham, 3 oz.	142	15.7	8.5	0.4
ham loaf, glazed, 3½ oz.	247	13.3	14.7	14.3
loin chop, lean, 1	170	23.5	7.7	0
fresh picnic, lean, 3½ oz.	150	19.4	7.4	0
sweet & sour, 7 oz.	386	19.1	21.7	28.7
sausage, brown & serve, 1 oz.	118	4.6	10.6	0.8
sausage, fresh link, ½ oz.	48	2.6	4.1	0.1
sausage, fresh patty, 1 oz.	100	5.3	8.4	0.3
Pork & beef, fresh link, 1, ½ oz.	52	1.8	4.7	0.4
spareribs, 3 med. roasted	198	9.4	17.5	0
tenderloin, lean roasted, 3½ oz.	239	30.6	12.1	0
Potato, long type, 4¾-inch	143	13.9	0.2	32.1
round, 2½-inch	86	2.4	0.1	19.2
boiled, 1 cup diced	118	3.3	0.2	26.5
mashed, 1 cup	137	4.4	1.5	27.3
french fried, 10 fries	214	3.4	10.3	28.1
chips, 1 oz.	161	1.5	11.3	14.2
Potato salad, 1 cup	363	7.5	23	33.5
Prunes, 10 dried w/o pits	260	2.1	0.6	68.7
cooked w/sugar, 1 cup	504	3.4	0.6	131.9
dried chopped, 1 cup	408	3.4	1	107.8
juice, 1 cup	197	1	0.3	48.6
Pretzel, 3 ring, 10	117	2.9	1.4	22.8
logs, 3-inch, 10	195	4.9	2.3	38
rods, 7½ × ½-inch long, 1	55	1.4	0.6	10.6

FOOD	CALORIES	PROTEIN (g)	FAT (g)	CARBO-HYDRATE (g)
sticks, 3, 2¼ × ⅛-inch	23	0.6	0.3	4.6
Pumpkin seeds, 1 oz.	155	8.1	13.1	4.2
Pumpkin, canned, ⅖ cup	33	0.9	0.3	7.9
Rabbit, baked, 3½ oz.	177	30.9	5	0
stewed, 3½ oz.	216	29.3	10.1	0
Raccoon, roasted, 3½ oz.	255	29.2	14.5	0
Radish, 10 medium	8	0.5	tr	1.6
Raisins, 1 cup	419	3.6	0.3	112
1 tbs.	26	0.2	tr	7
Raspberries, fresh black,				
1 cup	98	2	1.9	21
1 cup red	70	1.5	0.6	16.7
Rice, brown, 1 cup cooked	232	4.9	1.2	49.7
white, 1 cup cooked	223	4.1	0.2	49.6
pudding w/raisins, 1 cup	387	9.5	8.2	70.8
Rolls, 3¾-inch hard	156	4.9	1.6	29.8
brown & serve	92	2.4	2.2	15.3
butterflake, canned	110	3	3	17
butterfly, Sara Lee	105	2.6	4.2	14.3
buttermilk from mix	113	2	4.9	14.8
buttermilk, Wonder	84	2.2	2.5	12.4
cloverleaf, 2½-inch	83	2.3	1.6	14.8
crescent, canned dough	100	2	5	12
croissant, Sara Lee	109	2.3	6.1	11.2
dinner/pan roll	85	2.4	2.1	14
finger, Sara Lee	59	1.6	2.1	8.3
French	137	4.3	0.4	28.3
gem style, Wonder	80	2.2	2.2	12.7
hamburger	114	3.4	2.1	20.1
hot dog	116	3.4	2.1	21
kaiser, small roll	93	3	1.8	16
parkerhouse, 2½-inch	75	2.1	1.4	13.3
rye roll	55	1.4	1.6	8.6
dark rye hard roll	80	3.1	1	14.6
sandwich roll	162	5.3	3.1	27.9
sesame seed roll	59	1.6	2.1	8.3
wheat roll	52	1.3	1.7	7.9
Rye flour, 1 cup	364	9.6	1	79.5

FOOD	CALORIES	PROTEIN (g)	FAT (g)	CARBO-HYDRATE (g)
Salad dressing, 1 tbs., blue cheese	76	0.7	7.8	1.1
French	66	0.1	6.2	2.8
Italian	83	tr	9	1
Thousand Island	80	0.1	2.5	2
diet blue cheese	12	0.5	0.9	0.7
diet French	15	0.1	0.7	2.5
diet Italian	8	tr	0.7	0.4
Sardines, Pacific raw, 3½ oz.	160	19.2	8.6	0
in brine, 3½ oz.	196	18.8	12	1.7
in mustard sauce, 1 can	230	18	17	0
in soy sauce, 1 can	380	18	34	0
in tomato sauce, 1 can	230	18	17	0.8
Sauerkraut, 1 cup	42	2.4	0.5	9.4
Sausage, cold cut bologna, 1 oz.	86	3.4	7.8	0.3
liverwurst, 1 oz.	66	5.4	4.8	0
blood sausage, 1 oz.	95	3.7	8.6	0.3
bratwurst, 3 oz.	256	12	22	1.8
chorizo, 2 oz.	265	14.5	23	0
frankfurter, beef	145	5.1	13.2	1.1
chicken	116	5.8	8.8	3.1
corn dog	330	10	20	27.3
pork & beef w/cheese	145	5.4	13.5	0.7
turkey	100	5.8	8.1	2.7
mortadella, 1 slice	47	2.5	3.8	0.5
olive loaf, 1 slice	67	3.4	4.7	2.6
pepperoni, 1 slice	27	1.2	2.4	0.2
salami, beef, 1 slice	58	3.4	4.6	0.6
deviled ham, ½ can	220	9	20	1
potted meat, 2 oz.	115	7.9	8.8	0.5
Spam, 1 oz.	87	3.9	7.4	1.1
thuringer/cervelat, 1	70	3.4	6.2	0.7
vienna sausage	45	1.7	4	0.3
Scallops, bay, raw, 3½ oz.	81	15.3	0.4	3.3
steamed, 3½ oz.	112	23.2	1.4	1.8
breaded & fried, 3½ oz.	194	18	10.5	8.4

FOOD	CALORIES	PROTEIN (g)	FAT (g)	CARBO-HYDRATE (g)
Sesame seeds, 1 tbs.	47	1.5	4.3	1.4
Sherbet, orange, 1 cup	270	2.2	3.8	58.7
homemade lemon, ¾ cup	241	5	5.4	44.9
other flavors, 1 cup	236	2.8	0	57.6
Shortening, 1 tbs.	106	0	12	0
Snail, raw, 3½ oz.	90	16.1	1.4	2
giant African, 3½ oz.	73	9.9	1.4	4.4
Soup, commercial, 1 cup,				
beef broth	64	10.3	0	5.4
chicken consommé	44	6.9	0.2	3.7
asparagus, cream	161	6.3	8.2	16.4
bean w/bacon	173	7.9	5.9	22.8
bean w/frank	187	10	7	22
beef noodle	84	4.8	3.1	9
black bean	116	5.6	1.5	19.8
cream of celery	165	5.7	9.7	14.5
chicken & dumpling	97	5.6	5.5	6
chunky chicken	178	12.7	6.6	17.3
cream of chicken	191	7.5	11.5	15
chicken gumbo	56	2.6	1.4	8.4
chicken noodle	75	4	2.5	9.4
chicken rice	60	3.5	1.9	7.2
chili beef	169	6.7	6.6	21.5
Manhattan clam chowder	78	4.2	2.3	12.2
New England chowder	163	9.5	6.6	16.6
gazpacho	57	8.7	2.2	0.8
minestrone	83	4.3	2.5	11.2
mushroom cream	203	6.1	13.6	15
onion	57	3.8	1.7	8.2
oyster stew	134	6.1	7.9	9.8
potato cream	148	5.8	6.5	17.2
shrimp cream	165	6.8	9.3	13.9
tomato cream	160	6.1	6	22.3
tomato rice	120	2.1	2.7	21.9
turkey noodle	69	3.9	2	8.6
vegetable beef	79	5.6	1.9	10.2
Soybean curd (tofu), 2½ ×				
2½ × 1-inch	86	9.4	5	2.9

FOOD	CALORIES	PROTEIN (g)	FAT (g)	CARBO-HYDRATE (g)
Soybean flour, 1 cup	358	31.2	17.3	25.8
Spaghetti, 2 oz. dry	209	7	0.6	42.8
Spinach, 1 cup cooked	41	5.4	0.5	6.5
1 cup raw	14	1.8	0.2	2.4
Squash, acorn baked, ½	86	3	0.2	21.8
acorn mashed, 1 cup	83	2.9	0.2	20.6
butternut mashed, 1 cup	139	3.7	0.2	35.9
hubbard mashed, 1 cup	74	2.7	0.7	16.9
zucchini, 1 cup raw	38	2.2	0.2	8.4
cooked, 1 cup	28	1.8	0.2	6.2
Strawberries, 1 cup whole	55	1	0.7	12.5
frozen sweetened, 1 cup	235	1	0.5	59.9
Succotash (corn & lima beans), 1 cup cooked	158	7.1	0.5	34.9
Sugar, white, 1 tbs.	46	0	0	11.9
1 cup	770	0	0	199
brown, 1 tbs. packed	51	0	0	13.2
1 cup packed	821	0	0	212.1
powdered, 1 tbs.	31	0	0	0
1 cup sifted	385	0	0	99.5
Sunflower seeds, 1 cup hulled	812	34.8	68.6	28.9
Sweetbreads, calf, braised, 3 oz.	143	27.7	2.7	0
beef, braised, 3 oz.	272	22	19.7	0
Sweet potato, 5 × 2-inch baked	161	2.4	0.6	37
1 cup mashed	291	4.3	1	67
candied, 3½ oz.	168	1.3	3.3	34.3
Syrup, cane, 1 tbs.	53	0	0	13
corn light, 1 tbs.	57	0	0	14.8
corn dark, 1 tbs.	60	0	0	15
maple, 1 tbs.	50	0	0	12.8
imitation maple, 1 tbs.	55	0	0	14.6
sorghum, 1 tbs.	52	0	0	13.4
treacle, 1 tbs.	53	0.2	0	13.4
Tangerine, medium	39	0.7	0.2	10
small	33	0.6	0.1	8.3
juice, 1 cup	106	1.2	0.5	25.2

FOOD	CALORIES	PROTEIN (g)	FAT (g)	CARBO-HYDRATE (g)
Tapioca, dry (quick-cooking pearl and granulated),				
1 cup	535	0.9	0.3	131
1 tbs.	30	0.1	tr	7.3
cream pudding, 1 cup	221	8.3	8.4	28.2
Tartar sauce, 1 tbs.	74	0.2	8.1	0.6
1 cup	1221	3.2	123.9	9.7
Tomato, green raw, 4 oz.	25	1.2	0.2	5
ripe, 3½ oz.	20	1	0.2	4.3
boiled, 1 cup	63	3.1	0.5	13.3
canned, 1 cup	51	2.4	0.5	10.4
Tomato catsup, 1 cup	289	5.5	1.1	69.3
1 tbs.	16	0.3	0.1	3.8
chili sauce, 1 cup	284	6.8	0.8	67.7
1 tbs.	16	0.4	tr	3.7
Tomato juice, canned, 1 cup	46	2.2	0.2	10.4
dehydrated crystals, 1 oz.	86	3.3	0.6	19.3
cocktail, 1 cup	51	1.7	0.2	12.2
paste, 1 cup	215	8.9	1	48.7
sauce, 1 cup	75	3	tr	18
Tongue, beef, 3 oz.	221	19.5	15.1	9.3
calf, 3 oz.	145	21.6	5.5	0.9
Tortilla, corn, 5-inch	50	1	0.6	10
flour, 1 oz.	95	2.5	1.8	17.3
taco/tostado shell	50	1	2.2	7.2
Turkey, light roasted, 3 oz.	150	28	3.3	0
dark roasted, 3 oz.	210	20	15	0
ham lunch meat, 1 oz.	36	5.3	1.5	0.1
loaf lunch meat, 1 oz.	40	4.5	2.5	0.3
pastrami, 1 oz.	40	5.2	1.7	0.5
Turkey roll, light & dark, 2 oz.	84	10.3	4	1.2
light meat, 2 oz.	83	10.6	4.1	0.3
Turnip, 1 cup cooked	36	10.6	4.1	0.3
greens, 1 cup cooked	29	3.2	0.3	5.2
Turtle, green raw, 3½ oz.	89	19.8	0.5	0
green canned, 3½ oz.	106	23.4	0.7	0

FOOD	CALORIES	PROTEIN (g)	FAT (g)	CARBO-HYDRATE (g)
Turtle eggs, 3–5 eggs	115	12.6	6.3	0.9
Veal, arm steak lean,				
3½ oz.	298	29.6	19	0
blade lean, 3½ oz.	228	36	8.4	0
breast stew lean, 3½ oz.	346	27.9	25.2	0
cutlet round lean,				
2½ oz.	194	23.2	12.8	0
cutlet breaded, 3½ oz.	319	34.2	15	10.5
loin chop lean, 2½ oz.	149	24.6	4.8	0
rib chop lean, 2 oz.	125	19.5	4.6	0
rump lean, 2 oz.	78	15.9	1.1	0
sirloin, 3 oz.	266	25.3	17.4	0
parmigiana, 5 oz.	287	15.9	16.2	19.5
Venison, raw lean, 3 oz.	107	17.9	3.4	0
roasted, 3½ oz.	146	29.5	2.2	0
salted dried, 3½ oz.	142	31.3	0.9	0
Waffle, 4-inch square	140	4.7	4.9	18.8
Walnut, black, 1 cup				
shelled	785	25.6	74.1	18.5
8–10 halves	94	2.7	8.7	2.8
English, 1 cup shelled	651	14.8	64	15.8
8–15 halves	98	2.3	9.7	2.3
chopped, 1 tbs.	49	1.1	4.8	1.2
Waterchestnuts, 1 pound	276	4.9	66.4	14
16 medium canned	80	1.4	0.2	19
Watercress, 10 sprigs	2	0.2	tr	0.3
3½ oz. raw	19	2.2	0.3	3
Wax beans, fresh cooked,				
½ cup	22	1.4	0.2	4.6
canned, ⅔ cup	15	0.7	0.2	3.1
Watermelon, 1 cup pieces	42	0.8	0.3	10.2
1/16 of 16-inch melon	111	2.1	0.9	27.3
Wheat flour, 1 cup	400	16	2.4	85.2
bread flour, 1 cup				
unsifted	500	16.2	1.5	102.3
cake, sifted 1 cup	349	7.2	0.8	76.2
Whey, fluid, 1 cup	64	2.2	0.7	12.5
dried, 1 pound	1583	58.5	0.7	5
White sauce, thin, 1 cup	303	9.8	21.8	18

FOOD	CALORIES	PROTEIN (g)	FAT (g)	CARBO-HYDRATE (g)
medium, 1 cup	405	9.8	31.3	22
thick, 1 cup	495	10	39	27.5
Wild rice raw, 1 cup	565	22.6	1.1	120.5
Yam, 1 cup cooked	210	4.8	0.4	48.2
Yeast, baker's, 1 pkg.	15	2	0.1	2
Yogurt, whole milk, 1 cup	152	7.4	8.3	12
low-fat, plain, 1 cup	123	8.3	4.2	12.7
fruit flavored, 1 cup	225	9	2.6	42.3
Fast Food				
Arby's club sandwich	560	30	30	43
ham & cheese	380	23	17	33
junior roast beef	220	12	9	21
roast beef	350	22	15	32
roast beef & cheese	450	27	22	36
super roast beef	620	30	28	61
turkey	510	28	24	46
Burger Chef, cheeseburger	290	14	13	29
double cheeseburger	420	24	22	30
fish filet	547	21	31	46
french fries, small	250	2	19	20
hamburger, reg. chef	244	11	9	29
hamburger, big chef	569	23	36	38
hamburger, super chef	563	29	30	44
hamburger, top chef	661	41	38	36
hot chocolate	198	8	8	23
shake, chocolate	403	10	9	72
shake, vanilla	380	13	10	60
Burger King, cheeseburger	350	18	17	30
double cheeseburger	530	30	32	31
regular fries	210	3	11	25
hamburger	290	15	13	29
hamburger, whopper	630	26	36	50
hamburger, whopper w/cheese	740	32	45	52
hamburger, double beef	850	44	52	52
hamburger, double beef w/cheese	950	50	60	54
hamburger, jr. whopper	370	15	20	31

FOOD	CALORIES	PROTEIN (g)	FAT (g)	CARBO-HYDRATE (g)
onion rings	270	3	16	29
apple pie	240	2	12	32
shake, choc. or vanilla	340	8	10	57
Church's Fried Chicken, dark, 3½ oz.	305	22	21	7
white, 3½ oz.	327	21	23	10
Dairy Queen, cheeseburger	318	18	14	30
cheese dog	330	15	19	24
super cheese dog	593	26	36	43
chili dog	330	13	20	25
super chili dog	555	23	33	42
banana split	540	10	15	91
buster bar	390	10	22	37
dilly bar	240	4	15	22
hot fudge brownie delight	570	11	22	83
small cone	110	3	3	18
medium cone	230	6	7	35
large cone	340	10	10	52
small cone dipped choc.	150	3	7	20
ice cream sandwich	140	3	4	24
small choc. sundae	170	4	4	30
fish sandwich	400	20	17	41
fish w/cheese sandwich	440	24	21	39
onion rings	300	6	17	33
Jack in the box, breakfast jack	301	18	13	28
french toast	537	15	29	54
double cheese omelet	423	19	25	30
cheeseburger, jumbo jack	628	32	35	45
hamburger, jumbo jack	551	28	29	45
moby jack	455	17	26	38
taco	189	8	11	15
super taco	285	12	17	20
Long John Silver, chicken planks	457	27	23	35
clam chowder	107	5	3	15
breaded clams	617	18	34	61

FOOD	CALORIES	PROTEIN (g)	FAT (g)	CARBO-HYDRATE (g)
coleslaw	138	1	8	16
corn on the cob	176	5	4	29
fish sandwich	560	22	31	49
battered fish, 2 pieces	366	22	22	21
hush puppies, 3 pieces	153	3	7	20
scallops, 6 pieces	283	11	13	30
breaded oysters, 6	441	13	19	53
shrimp w/batter, 6	268	8	13	30
McDonalds, big Mac	563	25.7	33	40.6
chicken McNuggets, 6	314	20.3	19	15.4
egg McMuffin	327	18.5	14.8	31
fish filet	432	14.3	25	37.4
quarter pounder	424	24.4	21.7	32.7
Taco Bell, bean burrito	350	15.1	10.8	48.3
beef burrito	466	30	21	37
combination burrito	404	21	16	43
burrito supreme	457	21	22	43
taco	162	11.8	8.6	8.9
tostado	179	9	6	25
tostado w/beef	291	19	15	21
Wendy's single cheeseburger	580	33	34	34
double cheeseburger	800	50	48	41
triple cheeseburger	1040	72	68	35

Nutritive Value of Foods, Home and Garden Bulletin, No. 72. U.S. Department of Agriculture. Revised, 1981.
Nutritive Value of American Foods in Common Units, Agriculture Handbook, No. 456. U.S. Department of Agriculture. Issued November 1975.

General Index

[267]

DNA (deoxyribonucleic acid),
24, 35–36, 38, 45, 214,
219
  mutations, 208
  regulation of body pro-
  cesses, 35–36

Ears, ringing in, 213
Eating behavior
  endorphins, 199
  evaluation of, 201
  lack of self-discipline, 187–
  89
  metabolism and, 178–79
  social event, 203
  stress, 199–201
  Ultrafit State and, 126
Eating games, 187–88
Eggs
  amino acids, 68, 82
  egg whites, 216, 229
  fat content and calories, 125
Electron microscope, 38
Emotional stress, 1, 32, 43,
199–202
Endorphins, 173, 199
Energy, 4, 39
  production of, 37
Enthusiasm, 190, 194, 198
Enzymes, 38, 67
Equipment, exercise, 180
Esophagus, medical disorders,
78
Estrogen, 24, 37, 179, 182
  fat-related diseases, 22
  inactive forms of, 24
  muscle-building exercises,
  36–37
Evolution, 24, 28, 45
Exercise programs, 1, 4–5, 15,
19, 43–44, 58, 170–83

advantages of, 43, 180–81
aerobic vs. anaerobic, 82,
173–74
Amino Acid Diet, 10, 79
before and after meals, 182
blood pressure levels, 172
bodybuilding, 4, 60
buddy system, 181
to build muscle mass, 60,
182
calorie-burning rates, 175–
77
cholesterol levels, 172
dancing programs, 181
degenerative arthritis, 170
effect on metabolism, 52
effect on mitochondria, 35–
36, 38
energy needs, 10
equipment, 181
feelings of euphoria, 173
fitness centers, 181
hunger control, 183
to increase metabolism, 60,
172–77, 226
to lose weight, 20, 38
mood altering, 72–73
muscle building, 37, 60, 182
opposition to, 48
recommended, 180–81
Reducing Diets, 89
sleep and, 183
time for exercising, 181–82
as tranquilizer, 170
treadmill, 171
value of exercise, 170–73
walking, 171–72, 180

Family conferences, 49
Family history, 15
Family relationships, 200

Recipe Index